THE AUTHOR

A qualified exercise teacher, Rosemary Conley has worked in the field of diet and fitness for over twenty years, but it was in 1986 that she discovered by accident that low-fat eating led to a leaner body. Forced on to a low-fat diet as a result of a gallstone problem, not only did Rosemary avoid major surgery but her previously disproportionately large hips and thighs reduced dramatically in size. After extensive research and trials, her *Hip and Thigh Diet* was published in 1988 by Arrow Books. This book and its sequel, *Rosemary Conley's Complete Hip and Thigh Diet*, dominated the bestseller lists for over five years and have sold in excess of two million copies. Subsequent titles, *Hip and Thigh Diet Cookbook* and *New Hip and Thigh Diet Cookbook* (written with chef and cookery writer Patricia Bourne), *Inch Loss Plan*, *Metabolism Booster Diet*, *Whole Body Programme*, *Shape Up For Summer* and *Beach Body Plan*, have all been instant bestsellers.

Rosemary has travelled the world promoting her books and appears regularly on television and radio. Since 1990 she has presented her own diet and fitness series on network television and currently appears on ITV's popular *This Morning* programme. Rosemary has also released many fitness videos with total sales exceeding one million copies.

In 1993 the Rosemary Conley Diet and Fitness Clubs were launched across the United Kingdom. Operating under a franchise system, carefully selected instructors are fully trained to teach the Rosemary Conley philosophy. It is the fastest growing franchise operation in the United Kingdom, with classes proving extremely popular, fulfilling a need to give additional support to followers of Rosemary's diets. It is the first national diet and fitness organisation where only qualified instructors are in operation.

Rosemary lives in Leicestershire with her husband, Mike Rimmington, with whom she runs Rosemary Conley Enterprises and Rosemary Conley Diet and Fitness Clubs Limited. She has a daughter by her first marriage and they are all committed Christians.

Also in Arrow by Rosemary Conley

Rosemary Conley's Hip and Thigh Diet
Rosemary Conley's Complete Hip and Thigh Diet
Rosemary Conley's Inch Loss Plan
Rosemary Conley's Hip and Thigh Diet Cookbook (with Patricia Bourne)
Rosemary Conley's Metabolism Booster Diet
Rosemary Conley's Whole Body Programme (published jointly with the BBC)
Rosemary Conley's New Hip and Thigh Diet Cookbook (with Patricia Bourne)
Shape Up For Summer
Rosemary Conley's Beach Body Plan

Rosemary Conley's
FLAT STOMACH PLAN

ARROW

First published in 1994
1 3 5 7 9 10 8 6 4 2

© Rosemary Conley Enterprises 1994

The right of Rosemary Conley to be identified as the author of
this work has been asserted by her in accordance with the
Copyright, Designs and Patents Act, 1988

First published in the United Kingdom in 1994
by Arrow Books Limited
Random House, 20 Vauxhall Bridge Road,
London SW1V 2SA

Random House Australia (Pty) Limited
20 Alfred Street, Milsons Point, Sydney,
New South Wales 2061, Australia

Random House New Zealand Limited
18 Poland Road, Glenfield,
Auckland 10, New Zealand

Random House South Africa (Pty) Limited
PO Box 337, Bergvlei, South Africa

Random House UK Limited Reg. No. 954009

ISBN 0 09 948251 7

Designed by Roger Walker
Nutritional consultant: Penny J. Hunking SRD, PEA, RSA

Printed and bound in Great Britain by
Butler & Tanner Ltd, Frome and London

WARNING

If you have a medical condition or are pregnant, the diet and exercises described
in this book should not be followed without first consulting your doctor. All
guidelines and warnings should be read carefully, and the author and publisher
cannot accept responsibility for injuries or damage arising out of a failure to
comply with the same.

Contents

Acknowledgements   6

Read This First   7

Getting Started   10

The 28-day Programme   12

Recipes   156

Maintaining Your New Figure   180

Appendix

Fat Content Chart   181

Weight and Inch Loss Record Chart   186

Flat Stomach Plan Questionnaire   187

Index of Recipes   189

ACKNOWLEDGEMENTS

With the ever-increasing demands on my time I become even more grateful to those who help when the deadline approaches for the manuscript to be delivered. This book required a huge amount of work and would not have been completed without the willing and cheerful help of my staff. So a big thank you to my PA Louise Cowell for transcribing endless tapes of dictation and for all her help and encouragement. Thanks must also go to Emma Archer and Sally Jee for their help and cooperation. Special thanks also to Janet Thomson, Head of Training at the Rosemary Conley Diet and Fitness Clubs, for overseeing the exercises and ensuring that every workout will be safe and effective.

My thanks are due also to the many members of the Diet and Fitness Clubs who contributed their favourite recipes. The recipes were tested by a very special team of pupils at King Edward VII Community College, Coalville, Leicestershire. Many thanks to Lynne Peebles and her students for the energy and interest they devoted to ensuring that the recipes would be enjoyed by readers of this book. Thanks also to the National Dairy Council, the Kellog Co. UK Ltd and the Potato Marketing Board for their delicious recipes.

Special thanks must also go to the trial team recruited by ITV's *This Morning* who put the diet to the test. Their hard work and determination produced the most incredible results and provided the proof of the efficacy of the diet.

The unsung hero of any book is the editor. I have worked with Jan Bowmer on all my books since my *Hip and Thigh Diet*. Not only is she a very dear friend but she is extremely encouraging and supportive as well as possessing a great talent for editing my work into a popular format. Thanks are also due to Dennis Barker, Art Director at Arrow Books, and to Roger Walker, Text Designer. A book such as this requires a huge amount of effort to ensure that it is well designed and easy to follow. This could not be achieved without a hardworking and professional team. Thank you all so much.

Read This First

Would you like to be able to slip on a slim-fitting skirt or pair of trousers and stand sideways on to a mirror saying, '*That's* better, my stomach actually looks flat'? If so, then this book is for you.

I have received *so* many requests for a diet and exercise plan specifically designed to achieve a flatter stomach. It seems that, having sorted out the nation's hips and thighs, the persistent paunch is the next challenge! So here it is: a 28-day diet and fitness programme specifically designed to help you lose those inches from around your middle to give you back your waistline and achieve a flatter stomach. If you have excess weight all over, then you will lose weight all over, but I promise you that if you have a large stomach, this diet will certainly help to minimise the fat and reduce the inches in that area.

Tried and tested, the diet has *proved* to be incredibly effective. It worked for our trial team, and now it can work for *you*. (Full details of the trial will be published at a later date.)

First, we must understand the facts. If you have a large tum, it's because there's fat stored there. It's important to realise that you can't turn fat into muscle – they are physiologically different – so I am not going to ask you to do 300 sit-ups a day. Sit-ups will tone (strengthen) your abdominal muscles, but they will not get rid of fat. Instead, we are going to *burn* the fat from the body's fat stores through activity that will make our hearts beat faster and make us out of breath. This will cause the body to draw on its fat stores for the extra energy it needs. We

can also reduce bodies fat by following a low-fat diet, which has proved to be the healthiest way to lose weight. As the fat we eat deposits itself straight on our bodies, it is easy to understand that if we don't 'pay it *into* our fat bank' we can't 'put it on deposit'. Well, this all sounds very straightforward and logical, but the vital bit is putting it into practice and sticking at it long enough for it to be effective. That's where this book comes in.

Since I researched my Hip and Thigh Diet back in 1986, and following its subsequent phenomenal success, I have learnt a great deal about what people like to eat, what can be achieved through low-fat eating and what are realistic goals. Some people have achieved the most remarkable success. For instance, Maureen, who telephoned me while I was doing one of my regular phone-ins on ITV's *This Morning*, had lost 14 stone (101.6 kg) in 14 months by following my Hip and Thigh Diet. Another viewer rang to tell me that her father had lost 10 stone (72.5 kg) in 76 days on the diet and that he was now a new man. Nicole Blount, who appeared in my *New You Plan* and *Flat Stomach Plan* videos, lost eight stone (58.1 kg) in eight months. By using the same principle of low-fat eating and combining it with a specially designed exercise programme, you can make an enormous difference to the size and shape of your abdomen.

We gain excess weight because we eat too much, particularly fatty foods, and we deposit the excess as fat on our bodies. In some people

fat is deposited particularly on their hips and thighs, while in others it is deposited on their abdomens. Generally speaking, people fall into three basic body shapes: we are either pear-shaped, apple-shaped or heart-shaped. There is nothing we can do to change the basic shape that Nature gave us, but we *can* improve the level of leanness within our bodies and reduce the amount of fat. No matter what shape we are, once we are slim we will look terrific, so don't make your body shape an excuse for not trying.

I would never recommend that anyone aims for thinness, but if you do need to lose weight, then there is absolutely nothing wrong in getting slim. Being slim may not necessarily guarantee you will live longer or that you will be less likely to avoid disease, but what I *will* promise you is that if you *want* to be slim, and if you achieve your goal, then your life will be *so* much happier. Some people are overweight and happy. This book is not for them. It is written specifically for those people who want to make a real difference to the way they look and feel. It contains a constructive programme of activity that will greatly increase your *general* fitness and steer you towards a healthy-eating yet weight-reducing plan. You will find it easy to follow and so un-diet-like that no one will know you are dieting, and you will be able to continue to follow its principles in the long term without feeling any sense of deprivation.

Eating tasty, nutritious food is one of life's real pleasures, and we should never forget that.

I want you to stop seeing food as an enemy and start seeing it as a friend. Yes, you will need to make some changes in the way you shop and in the way you cook, but changing some old-established habits doesn't take long. Once you see those inches disappearing from your waistline and from around your abdomen, you will find the motivation to continue. This programme works just as well for men as it does for women. The end result will be a feeling of enormous satisfaction and excitement at the real improvement you can see, plus the added bonus of looking and feeling younger and having more energy and vitality.

So how does the programme work? It's now proven that low-fat eating is the most effective way of reducing body fat. The body's make-up includes bones, organs, lean muscle tissue, water and fat. We want to retain the lean muscle tissue and, if possible, increase it, retain the level of fluids that we need for general health, but *lose* as much of the fat off our body as is possible within the limits of good health. Muscle requires a high energy (calorie) input to maintain it, unlike fat, which requires no energy to sustain it. This is why an 18-stone (130.6 kg) weight lifter with huge muscles can eat vast amounts of food and remain large but lean, with very little body fat, whereas an 18-stone (130.6 kg) person with little muscle tone will gain weight easily on a relatively small amount of food. The more muscle tissue we have, the higher our metabolic rate. That is why the exercise plan in this programme includes a good proportion of muscle-toning (building) exercises. This will encourage the metabolic rate to *increase* and the lean muscle tissue that you already have to be maintained and increased slightly. Each day's workout will take you about 10–15 minutes. By practising daily you will be

amazed at your rate of progress and the difference it will make to your body. Set aside a particular time each day for these exercises and make sure you *do* them.

Over the last eight years I have received a huge mail bag and, apart from the many thousands of letters that I have received from people who have successfully lost weight on my diets, I have also gained many insights into the individual needs of dieters. As well as wanting to have a flatter stomach, many requested that they be allowed a treat later in the evening before they go to bed. There also appears to be a preference for a diet that tells you what to eat each day yet one that provides the flexibility of being able to swap around different menus to suit individual tastes and lifestyle. Taking all this research into consideration, I believe I have come up with the optimum package in this *Flat Stomach Plan*. The diet offers three meals per day, plus the option of an evening treat which can be the starter or the dessert from any dinner menu. The exercise plan incorporates a progressive programme of movements that work the whole body. As you become fitter, you will be challenged to work your body a little harder each day. On most days I have included an aerobic section to enable you to burn fat, and each day includes a toning section to enable you to increase muscle tone. By combining these two types of activity, you will optimise your inch loss and at the same time increase your metabolic rate.

Just as no one becomes overweight overnight, no one should expect to become slim instantly. In order to achieve a reduction in body fat you have to work at it and give it time to burn away. 'Quick-fix' diets have the effect of reducing the fluid level and lean muscle mass within the body, registering an artificial weight loss on the scales. Trying to lose weight by going on a crash diet is

as senseless as trying to get rich by gambling. It just doesn't work. By taking the time to do this 28-day programme, you will change your eating habits and learn how to work your body in a way that is safe and effective in reducing your body's fat levels and, at the same time, increase muscle tone. All I ask of you is that you make a commitment for one month and give this plan a real try. If you still have weight to lose at the end of the 28 days, the diet is perfectly safe for you to follow for as long as you wish. Just see the weight and inches continue to disappear. You can continue with the exercise programme by following the maintenance workouts available on video (see end of book).

It takes a month to change a habit and your eating habits are no exception. Make time for your exercises, then *see* the results. If you stick with this plan you will be so thrilled with your progress that you will find the willpower to continue to your goal.

I am often asked how we can drum up more willpower to stick to a diet or exercise plan. I have learned from experience that if you have a good enough reason for wanting to lose weight, you can definitely do it. So give it some serious thought and make a real commitment. Once you have made that commitment, and know why you have made it, it is much easier to continue. If you attempt to lose weight in a half-hearted fashion, making your own adjustments to the diet and trusting to luck that you are going to weigh less at the end of your campaign, you're wasting your time. All my diets contain calorie-controlled, fat-controlled menus that enable the body still to enjoy maximum nutrition and yet use up its reserves of fat. We also need to realise that there aren't usually *diet* failures but there are *people* failures. We blame a diet for not working when in fact the dieter cheats, fails and then blames ... the diet. I try very hard to make my diets as easy to follow as possible to ensure they are high in satisfaction and low in deprivation. You will only stick to a diet if you are happy with it, and you will only continue with an exercise programme if you start seeing results. They will work if you give them a chance, so please give me four weeks!

While we all hate having our photographs taken when we are at our largest, I ask you please to swallow your pride and ask a friend or partner to take a photograph of you before you commence this programme. We have very short memories when it comes to weight loss and we can so easily forget what we looked like before. If you have visual proof, you can always refer back to it, and this can encourage you to stay slim. Try on a tight-fitting skirt or pair of trousers before you begin the programme. Once you have started the programme, try it on every few days and feel how much looser it becomes. Never throw that garment away. Use it as a constant reminder for you to see how much weight you have lost.

Be realistic about your goals, and don't expect to be waif-like at the end of the 28 days. As I said earlier, thinness is not what we are aiming to achieve here. We are aiming to make a significant improvement to your stomach area and waistline as well as lose excess inches from other areas if necessary. Ask yourself this simple question: if you could lose a significant number of inches from your abdomen and increase the muscle tone in that area and indeed on your whole body so that you were a whole dress size smaller, wouldn't you say 'Yes, please'? You can make a dramatic improvement to your shape by following this plan, but it will require you to make some changes. If you are not prepared to make the commitment, I suggest you give this book to someone else. If you *are* committed, then we will work together to achieve the kind of body that you probably don't believe could ever be yours. Each day I will give you some encouragement and provide you with a menu that includes a variety of dishes from which you may choose. I will take you through a series of exercises that I hope you will find enjoyable and feel better for having done. At the end of each day I have included a 'positive thought' for you to consider to encourage you to continue to the next stage ... and the next.

Not all these thoughts are my own, but they are ones that I have learned and put into practice throughout my daily life. They make a big difference to my life and I hope they will to yours too.

Twenty-eight days is such a short period of time compared to the rest of our lives. By making a concerted effort you could make the most dramatic change in your life.

Since I am interested to hear of your progress, I have included a questionnaire on pages 187–188. There is no doubt that those dieters who feel that they have someone to whom they can report are likely to be significantly more successful than those who try to go it alone. Because of my ever-increasing schedule, I regret I am unable to answer readers' letters.

Getting Started

Decide on a day you intend to commence the programme. In the meantime, clear out the high-fat foods from your refrigerator and store cupboards and buy in only foods that are low in fat. Be imaginative with your choice of sauces and other cooking ingredients in order to enhance the flavour of the meals you prepare. With such a great variety of products now available in the supermarket there is no excuse to buy anything that is not low in fat.

Look at your favourite recipes and see how you can adapt them to low-fat eating. Instead of frying in butter or oil, get into the habit of dry-frying. Use cornflour mixed with a little water as a thickener instead of a butter and flour roux. Low-fat cooking is really easy, but you need to be imaginative and you need to experiment. Play around with flavours and textures and try different combinations of foods. Bacon enhances the flavour of baked beans, and Marmite eaten with cottage cheese transforms what some people would call a bland taste.

For added flavour I always use a stock cube in the water in which I boil my vegetables, rice or pasta. After cooking vegetables, don't throw away the water – you can use it to make some delicious low-fat soup. Take the trouble to make low-fat dressings for salads, or use low-fat brands. Add mint sauce to yogurt and use as a dip with carrot and celery sticks, cucumber and peppers.

Remember that calories do count, therefore if we are to lose weight we cannot simply eat endless quantities of foods that are low in fat. We need to eat sufficient calories to enable the body to have maximum nutrition and maintain its metabolic rate, yet at the same time control our calorie intake so that the body draws on its reserves of fat for fuel. It is a fine balancing act to maximise fat loss yet simultaneously increase our level of health and fitness. It is worth getting it right.

In the Store Cupboard

The following items are useful to keep in stock since they are common ingredients or accompaniments in low-fat recipes.

All-Bran
Arrowroot
Black pepper in a pepper mill
Branston pickle
Brown sauce
Canned mushrooms
Canned tomatoes
Cereals
Chilli powder
Chilli and garlic sauce
Cook-in-sauces (low-fat brands)
Cornflour
Curry powder
Dried low-fat milk
Fresh herbs and spices (any kind)
Garlic powder or low-fat granules
Ground ginger
Horseradish sauce
Lemon juice
Mint sauce
Mixed dried herbs
Mustard (French and English)
Pasta (egg-free)
Raisins
Reduced-oil salad dressing
Rice (preferably brown)
Salt
Stock cubes (beef, chicken, vegetable and fish)
Sultanas
Tomato ketchup
Tomato purée
Vinegar (including white wine vinegar)
Yeast extract

In the Refrigerator

Diet drinks
Diet yogurts
Fresh chopped vegetables (e.g. carrots, celery, cucumber, peppers and tomatoes)
Low-fat cottage cheese
Low-fat fromage frais
Orange juice (unsweetened)
Salad dressings (very low-fat or fat-free brands)
Semi-skimmed or skimmed milk
Sparkling mineral water

Utensils You Will Need

Non-stick frying pan with lid
Non-stick saucepans with lids

Spatula and spoons compatible with non-stick pans
Measuring jug
Garlic press
Chopping board and sharp knife
Kitchen weighing scales
Tablespoon and teaspoon for measuring

Cooking Tips

● Cook without fat at all times. Using non-stick utensils enables you to cook perfectly without it. Placing a lid on a saucepan or frying pan during cooking encourages more moisture into the dish being prepared and aids thorough cooking of the food.

● The flavour of some recipes will be further enhanced by allowing food to stand after cooking and then reheating before serving. Dishes such as kebabs benefit from marinating in a sauce *before* cooking in order to absorb maximum flavour.

● Always remove all skin and fat from chicken and meat *before* cooking to avoid the flesh soaking up the fat.

● Use low-fat yogurt in place of single cream in recipes, and low-fat fromage frais in place of double cream. However, never overheat these products or they will curdle.

THE FORBIDDEN LIST

Unless otherwise specified in the daily menus, the following foods are strictly forbidden whilst following the diet (some exceptions are made for vegetarians).

● Butter, margarine, Flora, Gold, Gold Lowest, Delight, Outline or any similar products.
● Cream, soured cream, whole milk, Gold Top, etc.
● Lard, oil (all kinds), dripping, suet, etc. (Vegetarians may use 1 teaspoonful of oil for cooking.)
● Milk puddings of any kind.
● Fried foods of any kind (except dry-fried).
● Fat or skin from all meat, poultry, etc.
● All cheese, except low-fat cottage cheese.
● Egg yolk (the whites may be eaten freely), except where included in a recipe or menu (although vegetarians should limit their consumption to 3 a week and non-vegetarians to 1 a week).
● All nuts except chestnuts.
● Sunflower seeds.
● Goose and all fatty meats.

● Meats products, e.g. Scotch eggs, pork pie, faggots, black pudding, haggis, liver sausage, pâté.
● All types of sausages and salami.
● All sauces containing creams or whole milk or eggs, e.g. salad dressing, mayonnaise, French dressing, parsley sauce, cheese sauce, Hollandaise sauce.
● Cakes, sweet biscuits, pastries (including savoury pastries), sponge puddings, etc.
● Chocolate, toffees, fudge, caramel, butterscotch.
● Savoury biscuits and crispbreads (except Ryvita).
● Lemon curd.
● Marzipan.
● Cocoa and cocoa products, Horlicks, except very low-fat brands.
● Crisps, including low-fat crisps.
● Cream soups.
● Avocado pears.
● Yorkshire pudding.
● Egg products, e.g. quiches, egg custard, pancakes, etc.
● Ice cream made with real cream (e.g. Cornish).

The 28-day Programme

Well, this is it. You've actually made the decision to start on this plan that will improve your shape and help you feel healthier and fitter than ever before. I am asking you to make a real commitment to stick to the diet plan and undertake the exercises on a daily basis. If you do, I promise that you will be delighted with the results.

First, weigh and measure yourself and enter the details on the chart on page 186. Make a point of weighing and measuring yourself at the same time each week, first thing in the morning before you eat or drink anything and preferably without clothes, in order to achieve the most accurate reading.

Initially, I want you to commit yourself to seven days of diet and exercise. Read the introduction and the positive thought for each day. I hope these will encourage you to stay on the right track and give you some interesting bits of information along the way. For the next seven days, I don't want you to cheat once, but I do want you to feel positive about your chances of success. If you want to lose weight badly enough, you can do it. Just follow the diet, do the exercises, don't cheat, and you will see the new, slimmer you emerging.

Remember to take some 'before' photographs of yourself before starting the programme. Take a front view and a side view. There is no need to show them to anyone until after you have achieved your goal. Take another photograph after 28 days and just see the difference. You will then be really pleased you took the trouble to record your progress in this way. These photographs will become your proudest possessions in months to come.

Finally, don't forget that skirt or pair of trousers. Try it on and feel how tight it is. Don't actually wear it for the next month, but keep it handy so that you can try it on every few days to check your progress. Scales can be deceiving because fluid levels in the body vary so much. However, inch losses that are witnessed by a swivelling skirt or a loose pair of trousers are genuine. Just think, at the end of 28 days your stomach is going to be significantly flatter than it is now. Are you prepared to make some sacrifices and go for it? Of course you are. You've got nothing to lose but those inches. Best of luck!

THE EXERCISES

The daily exercise routines have been carefully designed to work the abdominal muscles almost every day and other muscles every two or three days to ensure a fully balanced workout for your body.

Each day's workout commences with some mobilising movements to warm up the joints and prepare your body for exercise. These will minimise the risk of discomfort or damage and enhance the benefit of the moves that follow.

In preparation for the aerobic workout we perform two or three leg stretches to prevent muscle soreness. It is important that you do not rush these stretches.

The stretches are followed by the aerobic section, which consists of a low-level workout to raise your heart rate, improve your cardiovascular system and burn fat.

We then proceed to the toning exercises designed to benefit specific muscle groups, encouraging these muscles to strengthen and grow and resulting in a higher metabolic rate and an infinitely more attractive shape. The more muscle we have, the higher our metabolic rate, which is what every slimmer needs to achieve.

The toning exercises are followed by a series of stretches designed to encourage flexibility and enable us to maintain a full range of movement. These stretches also allow the muscles that have been worked to return to their normal physiological state, thus preventing discomfort. You should not feel any aches after your daily workout.

It is important to understand what exercise actually does for us. Aerobic exercise means any exercise which makes the heart beat faster. The heart beats faster because the body demands an extra supply of oxygen to sustain the activity. Breathing more deeply in the lungs allows us to utilise more oxygen and, in turn, enables it to circulate through the bloodstream to give us the energy we require. Aerobic exercise burns fat by using the fat around the body as additional fuel. We can continue aerobic exercise for a considerable length of time if necessary.

Toning exercises work in a different way.

These rely on the strength (pulling power) and endurance (staying power) of our muscles. Working a muscle strongly and performing a sufficient number of repetitions to allow it to become slightly fatigued causes that muscle to recruit extra muscle fibres, which increases the shape and size of the muscle. As muscle requires energy (calories) to sustain it, it is obvious that a person who has a high muscle mass will need more calories than someone who has less muscle and more fat.

For this 28-day plan, I have carefully worked out a series of exercises that combine fat burning with muscle toning to maximise the benefits as you reshape your body, giving particular benefit to the abdominal area. The exercises are progressive and should therefore be followed in the sequence laid out in the book. If for some reason you have to miss a day's exercises, it is important to return to that particular day's programme before moving on. Similarly, if you find some of the newer exercises too difficult, stay with the previous day's exercises until you become stronger and fitter and able to do the more advanced moves. To do a simpler version well and effectively is infinitely preferable to attempting a more difficult move and doing it badly. Only you will know if your body is able to cope. Listen to your body and if it tells you to slow down or that it's had enough, then take heed and just perform the stretches or have a rest. Do not overdo it. These exercises should not cause any physical harm, but if you feel any discomfort, stop exercising immediately and, if necessary, consult a doctor.

The exercises should be practised on a well-cushioned carpet. Alternatively, use a rug or foam mat to protect you from a hard floor. A sprung wooden floor is ideal, but try not to exercise on a solid floor. Always wear cushioned footwear for the workout, particularly the aerobic exercises.

Please do not rush your workout. The daily routines are going to have a dramatic effect on your body and your physical shape. Perform the exercises as described, and you will be staggered at the results. If you rush them and do them incorrectly, you will see little benefit.

Imagine you are doing the exercises in front of a panel of judges. Aim to perform each one perfectly, taking note of any teaching points in the instructions. Take your time and do only as many repetitions as feels comfortable for the aerobic and toning exercises. If you do not feel sufficiently challenged you will need to increase the number of repetitions. Vary the number to suit your ability. However, the stretches should be performed once only and held for 10–15 seconds.

If possible, exercise to your favourite music. This aids relaxation and you will be surprised at how much more you will enjoy the whole experience. The beat of the music will give you a momentum and enable you to continue for longer. Take the time to record your progress each day. Note how many minutes you worked out aerobically and jot it down alongside the last exercise that day.

Try to set aside a certain period of time each day for your exercise session. Ideally, perform them at the same time each day so that it becomes a habit. The rewards will be so great, you will be very glad that you did.

THE DIET

The diet in this programme is designed to give maximum choice to cater for every taste. There are quick and easy menus incorporating cook-in-sauces or simple cooking methods, as well as recipes for those who enjoy taking a little more time to prepare food. Select from the menus according to your purse, time and taste and the specific requirements of your family. This diet is suitable for all the family, but men over 5 ft 8 in (1.78 m) or who are involved in heavy physical work may increase quantities by 25 per cent.

The diet comprises two choices for breakfast and three choices for lunch and dinner, with the option of having a starter and a dessert *with* your main meal *or* saving one of them to have as a treat later. All the meals are interchangeable, so you can select any breakfast, lunch or dinner from any day. Your main meal may be eaten at lunchtime if you prefer.

Women are allowed one alcoholic drink each day, and men are allowed two. Do not save these up and have them in one go, as too much alcohol taken in one session will convert to fat on your body.

Do not eat between meals, but choose wisely from the menu suggestions and eat sufficient at mealtimes to satisfy your appetite and ensure any hunger pangs are prevented. Fill up on extra vegetables if necessary. If you feel really hungry between meals, then nibble on carrot or cucumber sticks. Do not eat fruit in between meals while you are on the diet, but you may do so once you have reached your target weight.

Ensure that all drinks are low calorie (these may be taken in unlimited quantities), and drink as much mineral or plain water as possible. Tea and coffee may be drunk freely, but I recommend you choose decaffeinated coffee and have your tea weak, as too much caffeine can be bad for us. Sugar contains only empty calories and should be kept to a minimum. However, a tiny amount taken in drinks will soon burn away and may prevent the temptation to eat sweet and high-fat foods such as biscuits, cakes and chocolate.

Potatoes and vegetables may be eaten in unlimited quantities with the main meals, but other carbohydrates such as rice and pasta should be restricted to a 2 oz/50 g (dry weight) portion. 8 oz (200 g) potatoes has the same calorific value as 2 oz (50 g) pasta or rice.

Diet Notes

Fruit
1 piece of fresh fruit means one apple or banana or 4 oz (100 g) any fruit such as grapes, strawberries or pineapple.

Yogurt
All yogurts should be low-fat, low-calorie varieties. Check the nutrition details on the carton to make sure you choose the right one. If it is difficult to find low-fat, low-calorie natural yogurt, try to select brands that do not have added cream.

Bread
Whenever possible, bread should be wholemeal. For guidance, one slice of regular bread from a large thin-sliced loaf weighs 1 oz (25 g). A slice from a large medium-sliced loaf weighs 1¹/₂ oz (37.5 g). Unless otherwise specified in the diet menus, 1 slice equals 1 oz (25 g). The term 'light bread' means low-calorie brands such as Nimble or Slimcea.

Sweeteners
Low-calorie artificial sweeteners should be used whenever possible in place of sugar.

Milk
Milk should be semi-skimmed or skimmed. Silver top milk is acceptable providing the cream is removed. Children under five should always be given full-cream milk.

Cottage cheese
Always select low-fat brands. Flavoured varieties are acceptable, but check the nutritional panel for fat content, and watch out for brands with added cream.

SAUCES AND DRESSINGS

The following may be consumed freely:

Brown sauce
Chilli sauce
Fat-free salad dressings
Lemon juice
Marmite
Mint sauce
Mustard
Oil-free vinaigrette
Soy sauce
Tomato ketchup
Vinegar (any type)
Worcestershire sauce
Yeast extract

The following may be used in moderation:

Barbecue sauce
Gravy (made with powder not granules)
Horseradish sauce
Pickles
Reduced-oil salad dressings (always use low-fat brands and avoid even 'light' brands of mayonnaise)
Sauces (e.g. parsley sauce, white sauce etc.)
Yogurt dressing

BETWEEN-MEAL SNACKS

The following may be eaten in moderation if you feel really peckish between meals:

Carrots	Celery	Cucumber	Lettuce
Mushrooms	Onions	Peppers	

Diet Instructions

Each day select one breakfast, lunch and dinner. You may save the starter or dessert from the dinner menu to have as a snack or small supper later in the evening. On the following pages you will find suggestions for:

BREAKFAST

2 choices

LUNCH

3 choices   Packed **P**

                   Quick and Easy **R**

                   Regular **Q**

DINNER

                   Starter

3 choices (main course): Regular **R**

                   Quick and Easy **Q**

                   Vegetarian **V**

                   Dessert

Daily Allowance

¹/₂ pint/10 fl oz (250 ml) semi-skimmed or skimmed milk
¹/₄ pint/5 fl oz (125 ml) unsweetened orange juice
2 alcoholic drinks per day for men
1 alcoholic drink per day for women

The following conversion rates have been used throughout this book:

1 oz = 25 g
1 fl oz = 25 ml
¹/₂ pint/10 fl oz = 250 ml

THE
28-DAY
PLAN

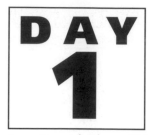

DAY 1

Today is a very important day. Weigh and measure yourself before you eat or drink anything this morning. Weigh yourself preferably without clothes, on a set of scales placed on a board to give the most accurate reading. Do not weigh yourself again until Day 8. Now measure yourself according to the instructions on page 186, and enter the details on the Weight and Inch Loss Record Chart. This is the first and most important step to a new body.

Are you ready to make the commitment? All I ask is that you select from the menu suggestions listed and follow the simple exercises that are illustrated on the next few pages. Do your utmost to avoid cheating. I would also ask you to be as physically active as possible throughout the day so that you get into the habit of being more energetic.

Acquiring good posture habits is vital in our campaign to achieve a flatter stomach. We often become lazy about our stomach muscles and allow them to just hang there. Through some effort and discipline over a period of days we can make a real improvement to our abdominal area. Our abdominal muscles act like a natural corset. Familiarise yourself with these muscles and use them to help you stand up straight by pulling them in as much as possible and as often as possible throughout the day to encourage them to become stronger. Look in the mirror and see the difference. People with good posture will often look younger than their true age and are less likely to have joint and back problems. There is no time like the present, so take this on as today's challenge.

Remember, the exercises in the aerobic and toning sections can be performed as many times as you feel able (although I have given an indication), and as the days progress you will be able to do more and more repetitions. However, the stretches should be performed once only and held in the extreme position for about 10–15 seconds.

Now, try on your tight-fitting skirt or pair of trousers and use this as your measuring tool to gauge your progress throughout the programme. Slipping it on every three or four days will give you a good indication of your inch loss, and you will be greatly encouraged as it becomes looser and looser.

Enjoy selecting your menus, and I hope you feel the benefit from the exercises. Stick rigidly to the diet, don't cheat, and you'll be amazed how quickly you will see the improvements. Don't forget, the menus are interchangeable from one day to another. Have a wonderful day!

MENU

BREAKFAST

¹/₄ pint/5 fl oz (125 ml) orange juice
1 oz (25 g) Bran Flakes, Fruit 'n Fibre, All-Bran or Bran Buds, mixed with 1 large chopped banana, and served with 4 fl oz (100 ml) milk (in addition to allowance), plus 1 tsp demerara sugar

or

6 oz (150 g) any stewed fruit topped with 5 oz (125 g) low-fat fromage frais or diet yogurt

LUNCH

Ⓟ Tuna Salad
2 slices wholemeal bread spread with reduced-oil salad dressing and filled with 3 oz (75 g) tuna (in brine) mixed with 1 tsp reduced-oil salad dressing, plus unlimited salad

Ⓠ 1 x 16 oz (400 g) can Heinz Big Soup plus 1 piece fresh fruit

Ⓡ Coronation Chicken Sandwich
2 slices wholemeal bread spread with 1 tbsp reduced-oil salad dressing mixed with 1 tsp each curry paste and low-fat natural yogurt and filled with 2 oz (50 g) chicken, 1 oz (25 g) raisins and lettuce

DINNER

STARTER
6 oz (150 g) grapefruit segments in natural juice

Ⓡ Apricot-glazed Chicken
(page 162)

Ⓠ Basil, Chilli and Chicken Stir-fry
(page 163)

Ⓥ Vegetarian Chilli con Carne (page 174)

DESSERT
Low-fat Trifle (page 178)

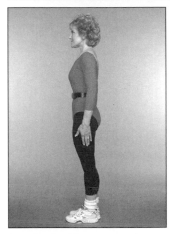

Start by checking your posture. Stand tall with tummy in and shoulder blades back and down. Try and maintain this stance throughout the exercises.

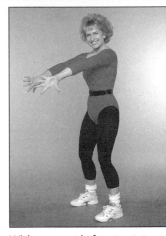

With arms out in front, rotate arms inwards and outwards. Do 8.

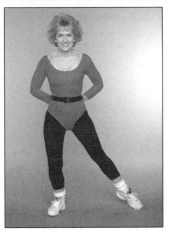

Extend alternate legs out to the side, tapping the toes on the floor as you step. Do 16.

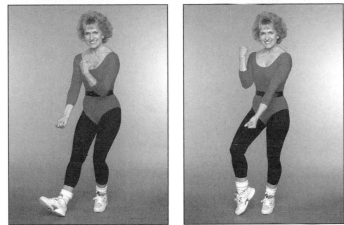

Tap the heel and then the toe of one foot, flexing and straightening alternate arms. Do 8, then repeat with the other foot.

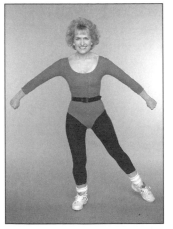

Extend alternate legs to the side, pointing the toes and swinging your arms in and out. Do 16.

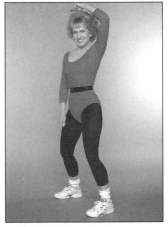

Rotate alternate arms backwards as if brushing your hair, transferring your weight from one foot to the other. Do 16

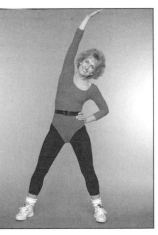

With feet apart, one arm raised and the other hand on your hip, reach over with the raised arm. Do not twist the hips. Return to the starting position, and repeat to the other side. Do 16.

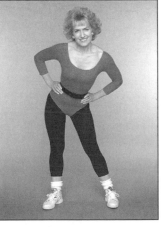

Rotate your hips in a clockwise direction. Do 8, then repeat in an anti-clockwise direction.

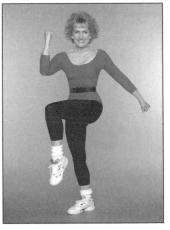

Raise alternate knees across and aim to touch with opposite elbow. Keep your tummy in and back straight. Do 16.

PREPARATORY STRETCHES

Back of Thigh Stretch Bend one knee and, keeping your weight on that foot, extend the other leg in front, toes raised. Feel the stretch at the back of the knee and the thigh. Hold for 10 seconds, then change legs and repeat.

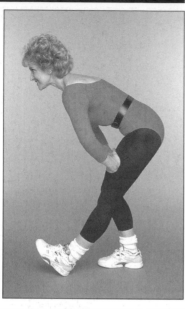

Calf Stretch Shift your weight on to the front leg and bend the knee. Your back leg is straight, heel on the floor and toes of both feet facing straight ahead. Keep your weight slightly forwards and feel the stretch in the calf muscle of your back leg. Hold for 10 seconds, then change legs and repeat.

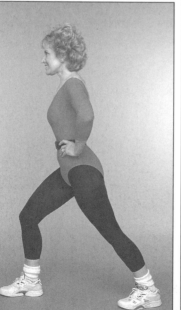

AEROBIC

Step and lunge to one side, reaching across with the opposite arm. Straighten the arm and the opposite leg as much as possible so that only the toes of that foot touch the floor. Repeat to the other side. Do 24 to alternate sides.

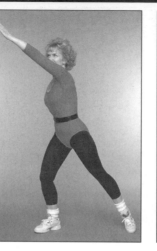

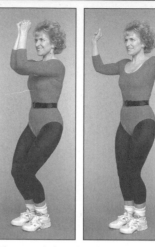

Alternately bend and straighten both knees, bringing bent arms in and out at shoulder level. Do 32.

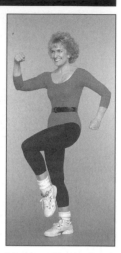

March on the spot, swinging your arms strongly. Don't stamp. Do 32.

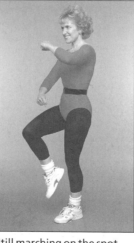

Still marching on the spot, beat an imaginary drum with your hands. Do 32.

Step back and curtsey, swinging your arms out and then in to cross overhead. Do 24 with alternate legs.

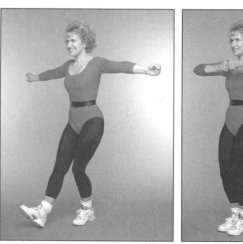

Tap alternate heels in front, swinging your arms in and out at shoulder level. Do 32.

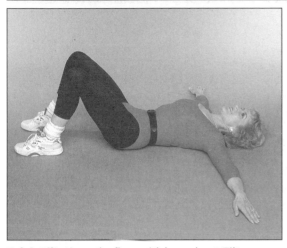

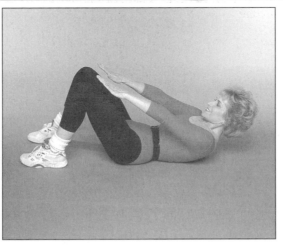

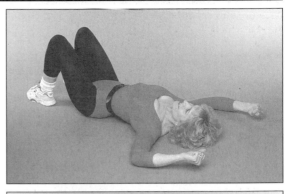

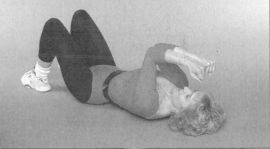

Pelvic Tilt Lie on the floor with knees bent. Tilt your pelvis forwards, pressing your tummy into the floor. Repeat the tilt 8–10 times. Remember this movement for all future abdominal exercises.

Tummy Toner Pull your tummy in tightly and gently raise your head and shoulders off the floor, reaching your arms forward. Keep a distance between your chin and your chest. Return to the floor, and repeat. Do 6–8.

Chest Toner Place your arms out to the sides, and bend them at shoulder level. Raise your elbows and press them together. Raise and lower arms 10–12 times.

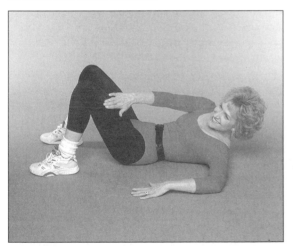

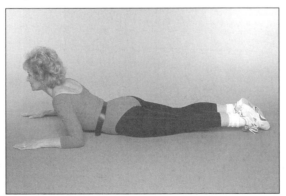

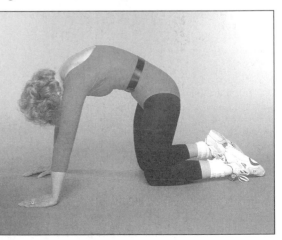

Waist Toner Supporting yourself with one arm, reach across your body with the other arm, pressing your tummy down as you reach. Take care not to roll the hips. Return to the floor, and repeat. Do 6–8, then repeat to the other side.

Back Strengthener Lie on your front with arms bent and palms down. Slowly raise your chest and shoulders off the floor, using the muscles in your back not your arms. Return to the floor, and repeat. Do 6–8.

Tummy Trimmer Position yourself on all fours and pull your tummy muscles in as tightly as you can to arch your spine. Relax, and repeat 6–8 times.

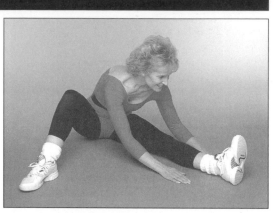

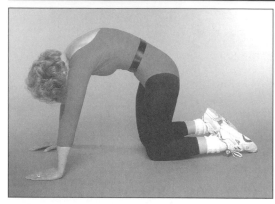

Back Stretch Still on all fours, arch the spine as much as possible, pulling your tummy towards your spine as you do so. Hold for 10 seconds.

Back of Thigh Stretch Sitting with one leg straight and the other slightly bent, ease your weight forwards towards the straight leg and feel the stretch at the back of the knee and the thigh. Hold for 10 seconds, then change the position of the legs to repeat on the other side.

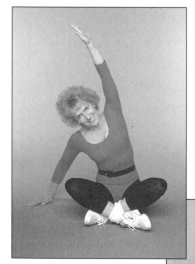

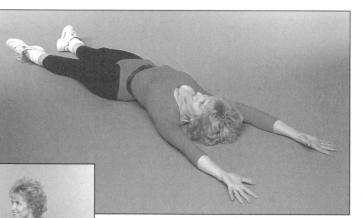

Waist Stretch Sitting with legs crossed, slowly reach over to the side with one arm, supporting yourself with the other arm. Hold for 10 seconds, then repeat to the other side.

Full Body Stretch Lie on your back and extend your arms and legs as much as possible. Hold for 10 seconds.

Chest Stretch Sitting with your legs crossed or extended in front (whichever is more comfortable), raise your arms and clasp your hands behind your back to stretch the muscles across your chest. Hold for 10 seconds.

POSITIVE THOUGHT FOR THE DAY

You have taken a very significant step forward in deciding to buy this book and commit yourself to the 28-day plan. Having read the introductory pages you are now well equipped to proceed to the next stage. Today you have started the diet and have completed the first exercise routine. This is a very major step and you are well on the way to success. If you continue with the plan over the next 28 days, I promise you will be extremely successful and delighted with the results. One of the most important elements in your success is developing a positive mental attitude. Do you feel in your heart of hearts 'Yes, this is it, I know this is going to work for me and I am jolly well going to do it'? Or are you saying to yourself 'This is just another gimmicky diet – I doubt whether it will work but I will give it a try for a few days'? If you have the first attitude you won't find problems, you won't find it difficult to cope when you are invited out for a meal and you will find a way of making time to do the exercises. If, on the other hand, you adopt the second attitude then, frankly, you would be better off giving this book to someone else. This diet and fitness plan will work beyond your greatest hopes providing you give it 110 per cent effort and determination. Isn't it worth making the sacrifice and commitment for just 28 days on the basis that at the end of it the results will be stunning? Those with a significant amount of weight to lose will need to continue beyond the 28 days and it is perfectly safe to do so. Remember, it takes a month to change a habit and the new habit that you will have learnt over these coming weeks will hopefully enable you to keep a wonderfully trim and healthy body for the rest of your life. You will have left those bad habits that made you overweight in the first place well and truly behind you. This diet will work for you but you are the only one at the helm. Please steer towards your goal.

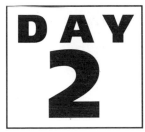

DAY 2

Did you enjoy the menus yesterday? Perhaps you were surprised that you were allowed to eat so much. The secret of any successful diet is that it offers plenty to eat so slimmers feel no inclination to cheat. Diets often fail because they offer too little food and slimmers overindulge in forbidden foods simply because they are hungry and feel deprived. Feel free to swap any of the meals for those from another day to suit your personal requirements.

I hope you managed the exercises yesterday and are looking forward to the next sequence today. Each day they become slightly more challenging which has the benefit of encouraging greater fitness, better muscle tone and increased fat burning. The more physically active we are the more we will increase our muscle mass which has the effect of *raising* our metabolic rate. At the same time we will decrease the amount of fat deposited on our bodies which will help us to feel fitter and healthier and will give us a more attractive physique. Strengthening our muscles will also help our posture. We strengthen our muscles by using them regularly and increasing the demands made upon them. The exercises within these daily routines are designed to do just that. However, unless you are a body builder regularly working with very heavy weights, you are unlikely to build a body that is unattractively muscular. What we are aiming for is a strong body with well-toned muscles. Muscle weighs heavier than fat and is also an active tissue requiring energy to sustain it. This is why the more muscle we have on our bodies, the more calories we need to sustain it.

In our everyday lives we often use our muscles, for instance in lifting children, carrying shopping, vacuuming or gardening. Look upon all of these activities as helping you to boost your metabolism and burn off some calories. *Any* activity is better than none. Enjoy today's exercises. Don't rush them, but take the time to do them properly. Feel your muscles working as you perform each activity. By doing the exercises correctly you will reap enormous rewards – but they won't be instant. So, be patient.

Enjoy today's menus. Select what you fancy, but don't cheat. Have a ·couple of long, low-calorie soft drinks prior to your evening meal and this will help you to feel fuller quicker. I always have two cans of caffeine-free Diet Coke before my evening meal and it makes an enormous difference as I have such a large appetite. It enables me to feel full when I leave the table, without overeating. Remember, quantities of vegetables are unlimited so fill up on these if you still feel peckish. I would rather you had a few more potatoes than three chocolate biscuits with the Nine O'Clock News.

MENU

BREAKFAST

¼ pint/5 fl oz (125 ml) orange juice; 1 oz (25 g) Bran Flakes, plus
1 oz (25 g) muesli mixed with 5 oz (125 g) low-fat natural
yogurt and 1 tsp honey

or

3 dried apricots and 10 sultanas pre-soaked for 12 hours in tea,
served with 5 oz (125 g) diet yogurt

LUNCH

Ⓟ Pork and Cranberry Sandwich
1 tbsp cranberry sauce mixed with 1 tbsp
low-fat natural yogurt and spread on to 2 slices
wholemeal bread.
Fill with shredded crispy lettuce and 2 oz (50 g)
cold lean cooked pork

Ⓠ 1 Heinz 'Lunchbowl' Country Vegetable Casserole, plus
1 piece fresh fruit and 1 x 5 oz (125 g) diet yogurt

Ⓡ Beefburger in Bun (page 160)

DINNER

STARTER
Crispy Garlic Mushrooms (page 156)

Ⓡ Chicken Dhansak (page 163)

Ⓠ Chicken Italienne
Allow 6 oz (150 g) chicken breast per person. Chop and dry-fry
the chicken until light brown. Add 1 x 14¼ oz (360g) jar of
Colman's Chicken Italienne Sauce (serves 4). Cover and simmer for
10–15 minutes or until the meat is tender. Serve with pasta twirls
or pasta shells (2 oz/50 g [dry weight] per person).

Ⓥ Spicy Chickpea Casserole (page 171)

DESSERT
4 oz (100 g) Wall's 'Too Good To Be True' ice cream
(any flavour)

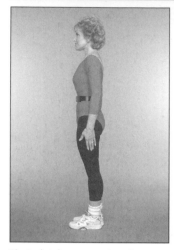

First, check your posture by standing up straight with tummy in and shoulder blades back and down.

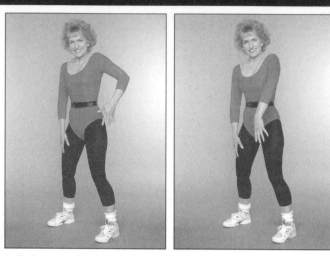

Roll alternate shoulders backwards, transferring your weight from one foot to the other. Do 16, then repeat, rolling shoulders forwards.

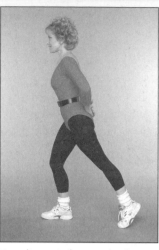

Tap alternate feet on the floor behind you. Do 32.

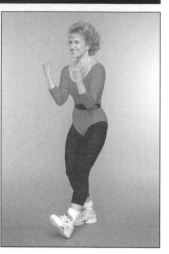

Tap alternate heels in front, flexing and straightening both arms as you step. Do 16.

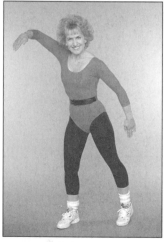

Circle alternate arms in a front crawl swimming motion, transferring your weight from one foot to the other. Do 16.

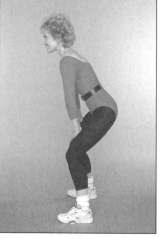

With feet wide apart, bend your knees and go down into a squat. Make sure your knees bend over the ankles. Come up slowly, and repeat. Do 8.

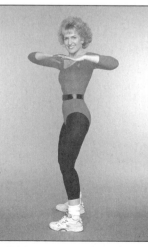

Keeping the hips square, twist your upper body from side to side. Do not jerk. Do 8 to each side.

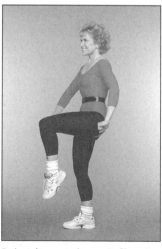

Raise alternate knees in front, pressing down with both arms. Keep your tummy tight and back straight. Do 16.

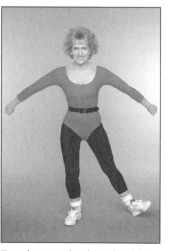

Tap alternate heels to the side, swinging arms in and out. Do 16.

PREPARATORY STRETCHES

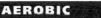

Back of Thigh Stretch
Bend one knee and, keeping your weight on that foot, extend the other leg in front, toes raised. Feel the stretch at the back of the knee and the thigh. Hold for 10 seconds, then change legs and repeat.

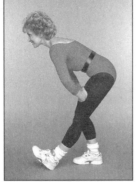

Calf Stretch Shift your weight on to the front leg and bend the knee. Your back leg is straight, heel on the floor and toes of both feet facing straight ahead. Keep your weight slightly forwards and feel the stretch in the calf muscle of your back leg. Hold for 10 seconds, then change legs and repeat.

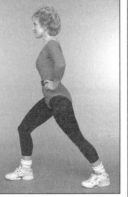

Front Thigh Stretch
Hold on to the back of a chair. Keeping your inside leg slightly bent, bend the other leg and take hold of your foot. Ease the foot back and up, keeping both knees aligned. Hold for 10 seconds. Release, then turn round and repeat with the other leg.

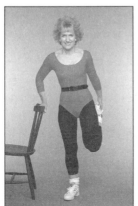

AEROBIC

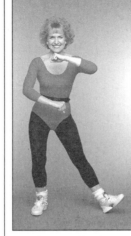

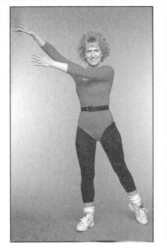

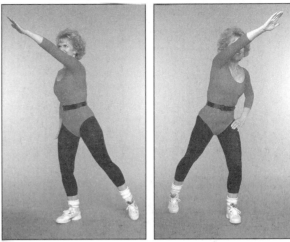

Tap alternate heels to the side, and beat an imaginary drum with your hands as you step. Do 32 with each heel.

Swing your arms from side to side as you step and touch the floor with alternate feet. Do 32.

Reach across with one arm and tap the opposite foot to the floor in a diagonal position. Do 24 to alternate sides.

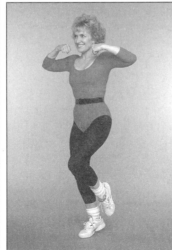

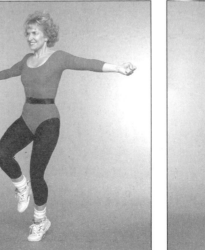

Jog on the spot, bringing your arms in and out at shoulder level. Do 24.

Raise alternate knees, bringing both elbows back to draw your shoulder blades together with each raise. Do 32.

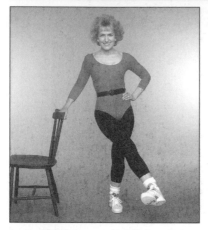

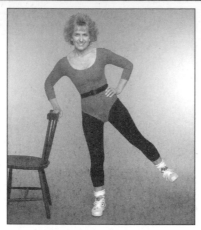

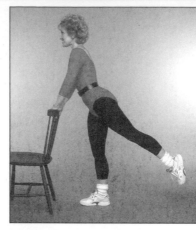

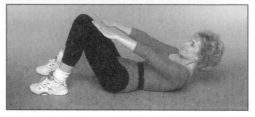

Tummy Toner Lie on the floor with knees bent. *Pull your tummy in tightly* and gently raise your head and shoulders off the floor, reaching your arms forwards. Keep a distance between your chin and your chest. Return to the floor. Do 10, raising on 2 counts and lowering on 2 counts. If you feel any discomfort in your neck, place one hand behind it for support.

Inner Thigh Toner Holding on to a chair, extend the inside leg forwards and across the body then back again. Keep your hips square. Do 10, then turn round and repeat with the other leg.

Outer Thigh Toner Raise the outside leg out to the side, keeping your hips square and toes pointing forwards. Lower the leg, and repeat. Do 10, then turn round and repeat with the other leg.

Bottom Toner Face the chair and raise one leg behind you, keeping the leg straight and squeezing your seat as you raise. Lower the leg, and repeat. Keep your tummy tight, hips square and your back straight throughout. Do 10, then repeat with the other leg.

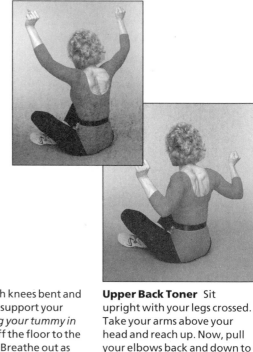

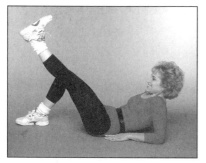

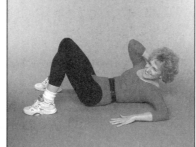

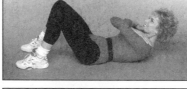

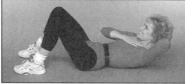

Front Thigh Toner Support yourself on your elbows. One leg is bent and the other is extended on the floor. Raise the extended leg to the level of the bent leg, then lower the leg. Do 8–10, then repeat with the other leg.

Waist Toner Place one hand behind your head and have the other arm on the floor for support. *Pull your tummy in tightly* and raise the head and shoulder, bringing the elbow towards the opposite knee. Take care not to roll the hips. Return to the floor, and repeat. Do 12, then repeat to the other side.

Tummy Trimmer Lie on your back with knees bent and hands placed across your chest. You can support your neck with one hand if you prefer. *Pulling your tummy in tightly*, raise your head and shoulders off the floor to the count of 2, then lower to the count of 2. Breathe out as you raise, and breathe in as you lower. Keep a distance between your chin and your chest. Do 10–12.

Upper Back Toner Sit upright with your legs crossed. Take your arms above your head and reach up. Now, pull your elbows back and down to squeeze your shoulder blades together. Raise the arms again, and repeat. Do 10–12.

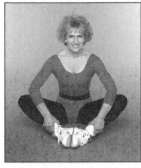

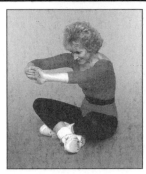

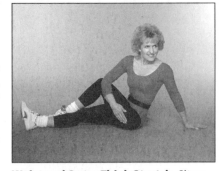

Inner Thigh Stretch Sit up with knees bent and soles of the feet together. Using your elbows, gently ease your knees down as far as is comfortable. Hold for 15 seconds.

Upper Back Stretch Still sitting with legs crossed, reach your arms forwards and round your back to separate your shoulder blades. Keep the arms at shoulder level. Hold for 10 seconds.

Waist and Outer Thigh Stretch Sit up straight with one leg extended and the other leg placed across it. Slowly twist your body away from the bent knee, using the opposite elbow to ease the bent knee further across. Hold for 10 seconds, then change legs and repeat to the other side.

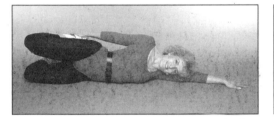

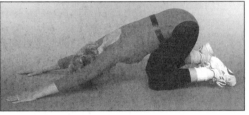

Front Thigh Stretch Lie on your side with both legs bent. Use your hand to ease the foot of the top leg back while keeping your hips square. Hold for 10 seconds, then roll over and repeat with the other leg.

Seat Stretch Start in the all fours position. Slowly ease your hips backwards without touching your heels and, at the same time, extend your arms in front. Hold for 10 seconds.

Tummy Stretch Lie face down with arms bent. Slowly raise your head and shoulders off the floor, supporting yourself on your forearms and elbows, and feel the stretch down the front of your abdomen. Hold for 10 seconds.

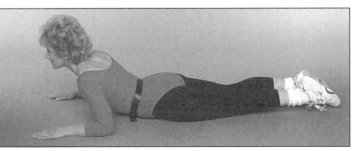

POSITIVE THOUGHT FOR THE DAY

How are you getting on? I hope you are enjoying the menu selection and are able to choose dishes that you really enjoy. Dieting doesn't mean starvation or deprivation. By eating nutritious meals three times a day we can eat really well. You are probably wondering if you will lose any weight when you are eating so much. Trust me, you will.

Yesterday your body performed a variety of exercises that it probably was not used to. You should feel better for it, and as the days and weeks progress you will find that your energy becomes greater and greater. Starting to take regular exercise is rather like opening a deposit account. The more time and energy you invest, the greater the energy return. You will be really surprised at the end of the 28-day period how much more energy you have and how much easier and less stressful life becomes. Exercise is truly magnificent in helping to alleviate stress and increases our sense of well-being. It will make such a dramatic difference to your body shape that the initial effort will soon prove worthwhile. Try to be as physically active as possible throughout the day in addition to following the daily exercise programme. For instance, park your car in the furthest space, not the nearest; take the stairs rather than the lift whenever possible and try to engage in sport, or play physical games with your children such as football or whatever. It will do the children good; they will think it's great that you are playing with them and at the same time it will burn extra calories. Look upon household chores as being part of your daily workout. Put that little bit extra energy into the vacuuming and realise how much energy you are burning off. If you have to clear out the shed or the garage, look upon it as a workout. All that lifting, brushing and general activity helps. Remember, the heart doesn't know the difference between physical activity involving a vacuum cleaner or doing an aerobic workout at your local fitness class. If the activity is making your heart beat faster it's burning fat. So from now on look at every physical activity through positive eyes.

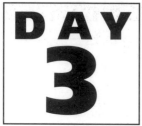

DAY 3

First thing this morning, slip on that skirt or pair of trousers to see whether they feel any looser. Hopefully, they will and this will encourage you to be extra vigilant today with the diet and exercises.

Today's exercises introduce some different moves which will further challenge your body. Increase the number of repetitions for the aerobic moves as you feel able and this will increase your general fitness. Try to do as many repetitions of the toning exercises as possible, resting if necessary between sets of repetitions, to enable you to reap maximum benefit. Obviously it takes a while for the body to adapt to physical changes but, believe me, it *will* happen and it will happen faster than you think. Perseverance is the key.

Prepare yourself a nibble box containing sticks of carrots, cucumber, celery, green and red peppers. If you find yourself feeling peckish in the evening, then nibble on these. The secret is to ensure that the food is prepared in advance. When we feel peckish, it is important to have an instant solution. If you don't have your carrot sticks to hand, you could end up having a slice of cheese and undo all the good that you have achieved over the last three days. Be prepared. Look out for the danger times and apply every shred of willpower you can. So many people when they follow a diet apply the 90 per cent rule. That is, they follow the diet and are good for 90 per cent of the time, but for 10 per cent of the time they cheat by nibbling, or finishing off the children's half-eaten sandwiches or leftovers from lunch. These little 'cheats' all add up to a significant number of calories to completely destroy the effectiveness of the diet. Yet people feel they are being *good* because they are eating the diet meals three times a day. Please don't fall into the 90 per cent trap. For this 28-day period make a pledge not to cheat. Those dieters I meet who tell me that they stick rigidly to the diet lose phenomenal amounts of weight. Why waste 90 per cent of your willpower only for it to be undermined by 10 per cent of unnecessary nibbling? Often the food that we nibble isn't even the kind we would choose to eat! It's just habit and pre-conditioning that drives us towards things not being wasted and the thought that 'one little bit won't hurt'. But *all* these little bits added together *will* hurt. Please don't do it.

Enjoy today's exercises and do them with extra vigour. Set yourself another physical challenge today too. In addition to your exercise routine decide on a physical activity that you can undertake for 10 minutes. It may be brisk walking, going up and down stairs, or working out to a fitness video. Choose whatever activity you like and, ideally, do it with someone else. Two people exercising together makes it more interesting, more enjoyable and you are likely to do it for longer.

MENU

BREAKFAST

5 oz (125 g) diet yogurt mixed with 1 pack any Kellogg's Variety Pack or 1 oz (25 g) any cereal; 1 piece fresh fruit

or

¹/₂ fresh grapefruit; 1 poached egg served on 1 slice (1¹/₂ oz/37.5 g) wholemeal toast

LUNCH

Ⓟ Oriental Chicken

Dice 2 oz (50 g) leftover chicken or turkey and mix with 1 tbsp reduced-oil salad dressing, a little low-fat natural yogurt, 1 tsp mango chutney, 10 sultanas, and chopped Iceberg lettuce. Place inside a wholemeal roll (2 oz/50 g) or 1 pitta bread or between 2 slices wholemeal bread

Ⓠ1 x 16 oz (400 g) can Baxter's French Onion Soup plus 1 slice wholemeal toast (no butter) and 1 piece fresh fruit

Ⓡ Jacket Potato with Fromage Frais or Cottage Cheese and Salad

1 medium (5 oz/125 g) jacket potato filled with 4 oz (100 g) low-fat fromage frais or cottage cheese, served with a large mixed salad (e.g. lettuce, spinach, bean sprouts, carrots, tomatoes, peppers); 1 apple

DINNER

STARTER
Carrot and Banana Cocktail
1 grated carrot mixed with ¹/₂ banana, sliced, and 10 sultanas and sprinkled with lemon juice

Ⓡ Sweet and Sour Pork (page 166)

Ⓠ Chicken Chasseur (page 163)

Ⓥ Stuffed Pitta Bread with Yogurt Salad
(page 172)

DESSERT
Tropical Fruit Salad (page 177)

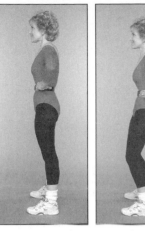 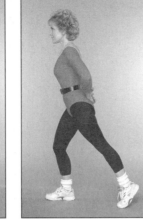

Stand in a good posture with your tummy in and your back straight, and tilt your pelvis forwards and upwards. Relax, and repeat. Do 8.

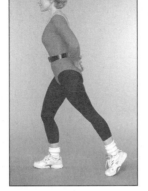

Tap alternate feet on the floor behind you. Do 16.

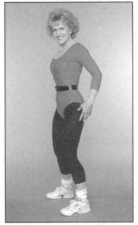

Roll both shoulders backwards while transferring your weight from one foot to the other. Do 16.

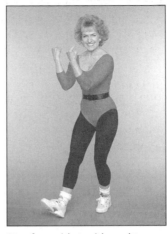

Step from side to side and tap the opposite heel on the floor in front, flexing and straightening your arms as you step. Do 16.

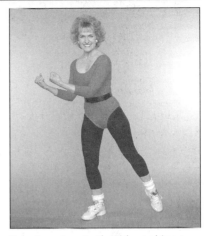

Take two steps to the side, making a scooping movement with your arms as if shovelling snow. Repeat to the other side. Do 16, alternating sides.

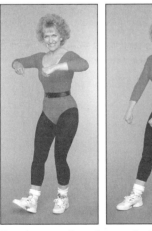 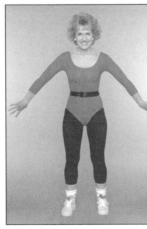

Tap the toes of one foot to the floor 8 times while punching down with your arms. Repeat with the other foot.

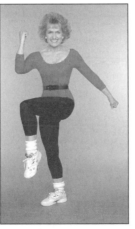

With arms out to the sides, rotate your arms forwards and backwards. Do 8.

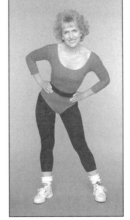

Raise alternate knees across and aim to touch with opposite elbow. Keep your tummy pulled in and your back straight. Do 16.

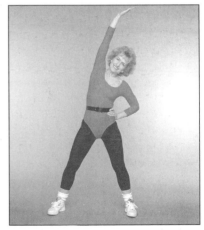

Rotate your hips in a clockwise direction. Do 8, and repeat in an anti-clockwise direction.

Stand with feet a comfortable distance apart, one arm raised and palm facing upwards and the other hand on your hip. Lean directly to the side without twisting the hips. Return to the starting position and repeat to the other side. Do 8, then repeat to each side.

Back of Thigh Stretch Bend one knee and, keeping your weight on that foot, extend the other leg in front, toes raised. Feel the stretch at the back of the knee and the thigh. Hold for 10 seconds, then change legs and repeat.

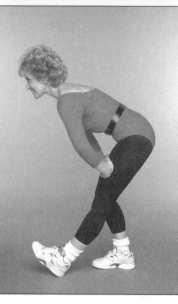

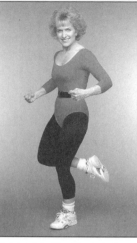

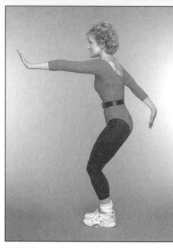

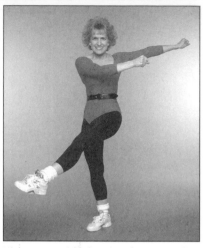

Kick back with alternate legs, bringing arms backwards and forwards as if pulling drawers out and in. Do 32.

With feet hip-width apart, bend your knees while swinging alternate arms forwards and backwards. Come up again and repeat. Do 32.

Kick across with alternate feet, swinging your arms from side to side in the opposite direction to your feet. Do 24.

Calf Stretch Shift your weight on to the front leg and bend the knee. Your back leg is straight, heel on the floor and toes of both feet facing straight ahead. Keep your weight slightly forwards and feel the stretch in the calf muscle of your back leg. Hold for 10 seconds, then change legs and repeat.

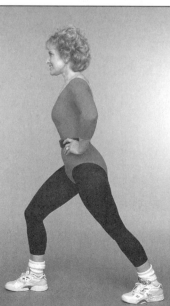

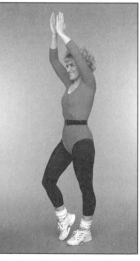

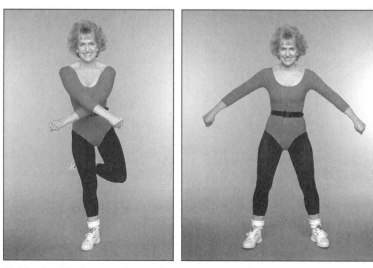

March on the spot and clap your hands above your head. Do 24.

Kick back with alternate feet, swinging arms in and out. Do 24.

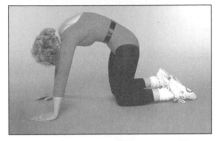

Tummy Trimmer Position yourself on all fours and pull your tummy muscles in as tightly as you can to arch your spine. Relax, and repeat 10 times.

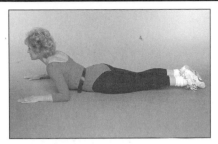

Back Strengthener Lie on your front and bend your arms, palms facing down. Slowly raise your chest and shoulders off the floor, using the muscles in your back not your arms. Return to the floor, and repeat. Do 8.

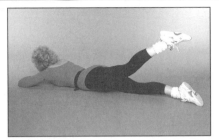

Bottom Toner Lie on your front with your head resting on your hands. Raise one leg straight up and down, squeezing your seat as you raise. Keep your hips pressed into the floor throughout. Do 10–12, then repeat with the other leg.

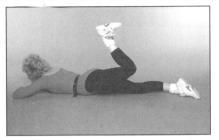

Back of Thigh Toner Still resting your head on your hands, bend one leg and push the heel towards the ceiling, extending the leg slightly as you do so. Do 10, then repeat with the other leg.

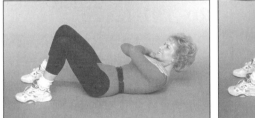
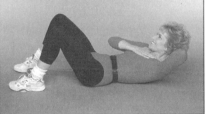

Tummy Toner Lie on your back with your knees bent and your hands placed across your chest. Support your neck with one hand if you prefer. *Pulling your tummy in tightly*, raise your head and shoulders off the floor for a count of 2, then lower to a count of 2. Keep a distance between your chin and your chest. Breathe out as you come up and breathe in as you go down. Do 10–12.

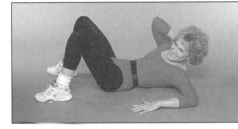

Waist Toner Place one hand behind your head and the other by your side. Raise your head and shoulder, bringing your elbow towards the opposite knee. Take care not to roll the hips. Return to the floor and repeat. Do 12, then repeat to the other side.

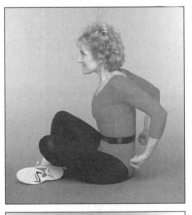

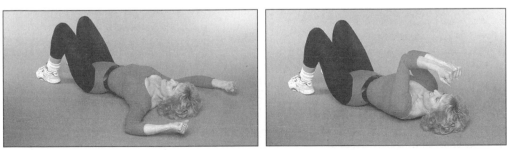

Chest Toner Lie on the floor with knees bent. Place your arms out to the sides, elbows bent and level with your shoulders. Lift your arms and press the elbows together. Lower the arms, and repeat. Do 12–14.

Upper Arm Toner Sit up with legs crossed, bend your arms and raise them behind you as high as possible. Keeping your elbows still, straighten your arms then bend them again. Do 12

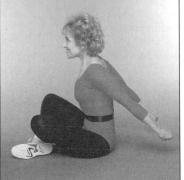

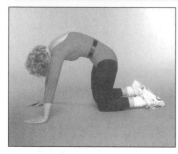

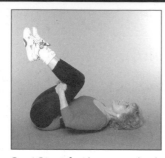

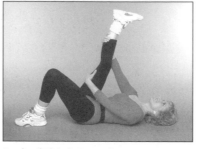

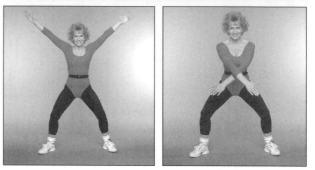

Back Stretch Position yourself on all fours and arch the spine as much as possible, pulling your tummy towards your spine. Hold for 10 seconds.

Seat Stretch Lie on your back with knees towards your chest and place your hands underneath your thighs. Ease your legs further towards your chest and feel the stretch in your seat. Hold for 10 seconds.

Back of Thigh Stretch Keep your legs bent and place the soles of your feet on the floor. Take hold of one leg and raise it, straightening it as far as is comfortable. Ease the leg towards you with your hands and hold for 10–15 seconds. Relax, and repeat with the other leg.

With feet wide apart, bend the knees and make sweeping circles with your arms to re-energise yourself. Do 24.

POSITIVE THOUGHT FOR THE DAY

By now you should be feeling that progress is being made. The waistband of your skirt or trousers should be a little looser, you should be feeling very virtuous having undertaken the exercises so far, and your body should be getting used to the fact that it is having a daily workout.

It is very important to be realistic about the goals that we hope to achieve. Whether we are a 'pear', an 'apple' or a 'heart'-shaped person, nothing in the world is going to change that any more than we can change our height. What we *can* do is improve the shape that we *have* as far as we possibly can and not underestimate what we *are* able to achieve. When I travel around the UK visiting the various Rosemary Conley Diet and Fitness clubs it is one of my most joyous experiences to meet members who have lost extremely significant amounts of weight and who have beautiful bodies to show for it. Bodies you would never imagine had been overweight in the first place. There has been so much research in recent years, and this has enabled me to come up with a really effective diet and fitness programme that I believe is the optimum in achieving the best possible results.

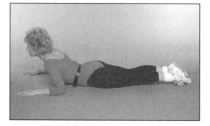

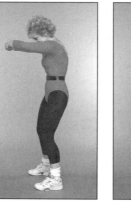

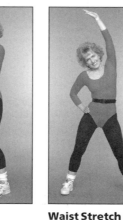

Tummy Stretch Lie face down with arms bent. Supporting yourself on your forearms, slowly raise your head and shoulders off the floor and feel the stretch down the front of your abdomen. Hold for 10 seconds.

Upper Back Stretch Stand with feet a comfortable distance apart and knees slightly bent. Round your back and raise your arms in front to shoulder level to separate your shoulder blades. Hold for 10 seconds.

Upper Arm Stretch Place one hand over the opposite shoulder and ease the bent arm across your body, using the other hand to assist. Hold for 10 seconds. Relax, and repeat with the other arm.

Waist Stretch Place one hand on your thigh for support and lean to the side as you reach the opposite arm over. Hold for 10 seconds. Slowly straighten up, and repeat to the other side.

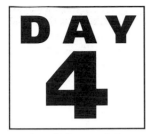

DAY 4

Well done for getting this far. Many dieters fail by Day 3 and the fact that you have reached Day 4 shows enormous determination and dedication. You are set to *win* and achieve this first goal and, by so doing, you will be making a very significant step towards improving your life in general and the way you feel about yourself and other people. In three and a half weeks' time you will see a dramatic improvement in your shape. You will be feeling so excited and proud that you have made the effort over these next few weeks. You are now over the first hurdle, so look forward with a very positive mental attitude. Don't make any excuses and don't look for problems.

Are you working on your posture and do you check it regularly? Make a real effort today. Start by looking in the mirror, notice how your tummy is reducing and your general shape is improving. Let this encourage you to make good posture practice a regular habit.

Make sure you eat your three meals a day and never skip breakfast. Breakfast is a very important meal and needs to be eaten to kick-start the metabolism. Failure to do so will mean that your metabolic rate will fall and you will find it harder to lose weight. Enjoy today's exercises and make sure that you play some lively music to help you along. Music can be very motivating and enable us to carry on exercising for longer than if we were to practise in silence. These exercises really will work if they are performed correctly and regularly and we need to make the whole experience as pleasant as possible. Enjoy today's menus and remember, no nibbling in between meals. Do have that long drink before your evening meal and have your nibble box handy if you feel you need it.

MENU

BREAKFAST

5 fresh plums plus 1 x 5 oz (125 g) diet yogurt

or

1 slice wholemeal toast with 1 tsp marmalade;
1 x 5 oz (125 g) diet yogurt and 1 piece fresh fruit

LUNCH

℗ Tuna or Cottage Cheese Sandwich

4 slices wholemeal light bread spread with reduced-oil salad dressing and filled with 2 oz (50 g) tuna in brine, plus salad, or 4 oz (100 g) low-fat cottage cheese and 1 oz (25 g) raisins or chopped dates, or 2 oz (50 g) cottage cheese and 1 mashed banana plus salad

Ⓠ 1 Golden Wonder 'Pot Light' Spicy Chicken, plus 1 x 8 oz (200 g) pot Müllerlight yogurt

Ⓡ Crispy Bacon and Beans on Toast

Chop a lean rasher of bacon into small pieces and dry-fry lightly. Add a little chopped onion and continue to cook gently. Add 3 large tbsp baked beans, mix and warm through.
Serve on 1 slice (1¹/₂ oz/37.5 g) wholemeal toast
1 piece fresh fruit

DINNER

STARTER
Grilled Grapefruit (page 157)

Ⓡ Spiced Turkey (page 165)

Ⓠ Stir-fry Chicken in Black Bean Sauce (page 165)

Ⓥ Tofu Burgers (page 172)

DESSERT
Apple and Blackberry Cake
(page 178)

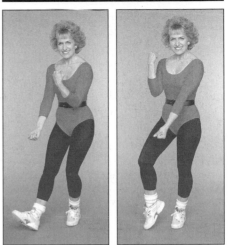

Tap the heel and then the toe of one foot, flexing and straightening alternate arms. Do 8, then repeat with the other foot.

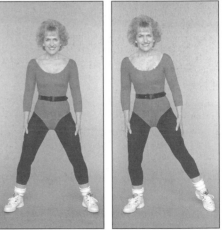

With feet a comfortable distance apart, transfer your weight from one foot to the other, bending your knees and tapping the toes of the opposite foot as you step. Do 16.

CONTINUED ▶

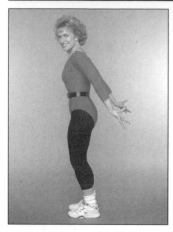

With your arms behind your back, rotate arms inwards and outwards. Do 8.

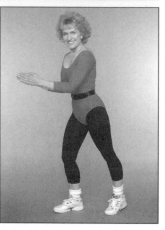

Rotate alternate arms backwards as if brushing your hair, transferring your weight from one foot to the other. Do 16.

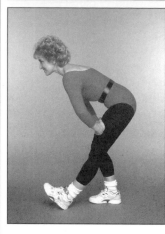

Take two steps to the side, moving your arms in a 'train-like' motion as you step. Repeat to the other side. Do 16 to alternate sides.

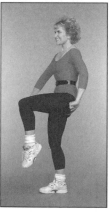

Raise alternate knees in front, pressing down with both arms. Keep your tummy tight and your back straight. Do 16.

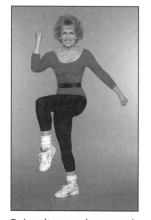

Raise alternate knees and aim to touch with opposite elbow. Do 16.

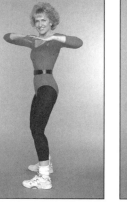

With feet a comfortable distance apart and arms at shoulder level, twist your upper body from side to side, keeping the hips square. Do not jerk. Do 16 to alternate sides.

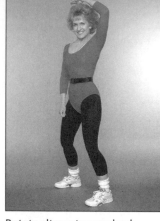

With feet wide apart, bend your knees and go down into a squat, making sure the knees bend over the ankles. Come up again, and repeat. Do 8.

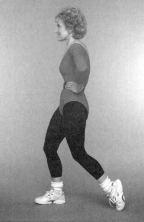

Back of Thigh Stretch Bend one knee and, keeping your weight on that foot, extend the other leg in front, toes raised. Feel the stretch at the back of the knee and the thigh. Hold for 10 seconds, then change legs and repeat.

Calf Stretch Shift your weight on to the front leg and bend the knee. Your back leg is straight, heel on the floor and toes of both feet facing straight ahead. Keep your weight slightly forwards and feel the stretch in the calf muscle of your back leg. Hold for 10 seconds, then change legs and repeat.

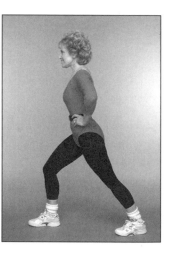

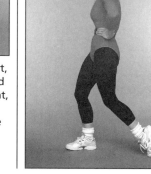

Upper Thigh Stretch Place one foot behind the other and, bending both knees slightly, push the hips forwards to feel the stretch down the front of the hip of the back leg. Hold for 10 seconds. Relax, and repeat with the other leg.

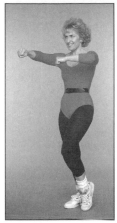 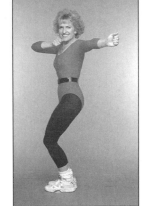 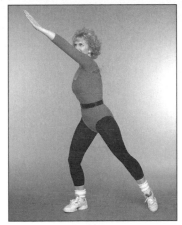 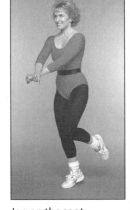

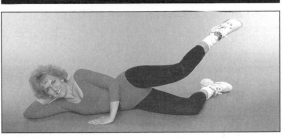

Outer Thigh Toner Lie on your side and bend both knees. Raise and then lower the top leg, keeping it bent. Make sure the hips are square and the knees and toes face forwards. Do 10–12, then roll over, and repeat with the other leg.

March on the spot and punch alternate hands forwards. Don't stamp. Do 32.

Bend your knees and pull an imaginary bow and arrow with your arms, then straighten the knees, and repeat to the other side. Do 24 to alternate sides.

Step and lunge to one side and reach across with opposite arm. Only the toes of the straight leg should touch the floor. Try to straighten the arm and leg as much as possible as you lunge. Repeat to the other side. Do 24 to alternate sides.

Jog on the spot, swinging your arms out and in and crossing them in front as you jog. Make sure the knees are soft and heels are down as you land. Do 32.

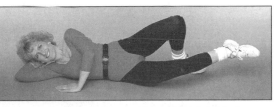

Inner Thigh Toner Place the foot of the top leg flat on the floor behind the bent lower leg. Raise the bottom leg as high as possible, keeping it slightly bent and making sure your hips remain square. Lower the leg, and repeat. Do 10–12, then roll over, and repeat with the other leg.

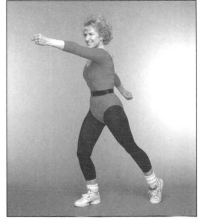 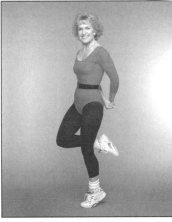 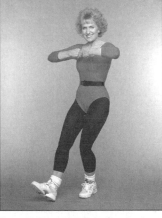

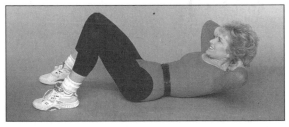

Step and touch behind with alternate feet, swinging alternate arms forwards and backwards. Do 24.

Jog on the spot, swinging your arms out and in to cross behind your back. Knees should be soft and heels down as you land. Do 24.

Tap alternate heels in front, bringing your arms in and out at shoulder level. Do 24.

Tummy Toner Lie on your back with knees bent and hands placed behind your head. *Pull your tummy in tightly* and slowly raise your head and shoulders off the floor for a count of 2. Keep a distance between your chin and chest. Return to the floor on a count of 2. Repeat 6–8 times, breathing out and you come up and breathing in as you go down

Chest Toner Still lying on the floor with knees bent, place your arms out to the sides with elbows bent at shoulder level. Lift your arms and press the elbows and palms together. Keeping the arms together and parallel with the floor, push them over your head and then pull them forwards again. Repeat this backwards and forwards movement 10–12 times, keeping the elbows together throughout the exercise.

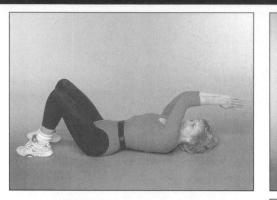

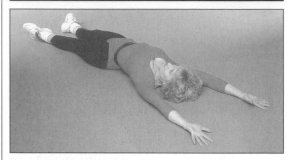

Full Body Stretch Lie on your back and extend your arms and legs as much as possible. Hold for 10 seconds.

Upper Arm Toner Bend your arms and place them over your head. Straighten the arms, then bend them again. Repeat this movement 12–14 times.

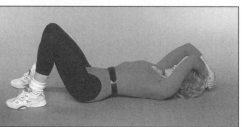

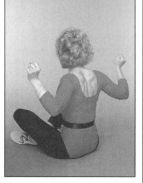

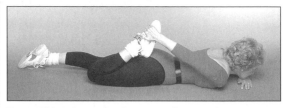

Front Thigh Stretch Lie on your front and rest your head on one hand. Bend the opposite leg and use your hand to ease the foot towards your seat. Hold for 10 seconds. Relax, and repeat with the other leg.

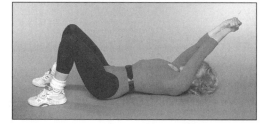

Upper Back Toner Sit upright with your legs crossed. Take your arms above your head and reach up. Pull the elbows back and down to squeeze your shoulder blades together. Raise the arms again, and repeat. Do 10–12.

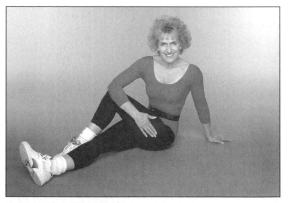

Tummy Toner Place your feet against a wall or on a sturdy chair, and support your head with your hands. *Pulling your tummy in tightly*, raise your head and shoulders off the floor, keeping a distance between your chin and your chest. Raise on a count of 2, and return to the floor on a count of 2. Repeat 10–12 times.

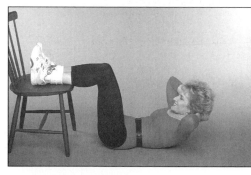

Outer Thigh Stretch Sit up with one leg extended and the other leg bent and placed across the straight leg approximately level with the knee. Use the opposite elbow to ease the bent knee across. Hold for 10 seconds. Relax, and change position to repeat with the other leg.

COOL-DOWN STRETCHES

Inner Thigh Stretch
Sit up with knees bent and soles of the feet together. Using your elbows, gently ease your knees down as far as is comfortable. Hold for 15 seconds.

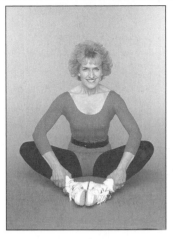

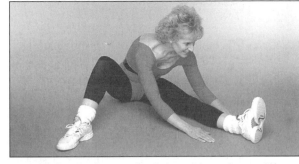

Back of the Thigh Stretch Sitting with one leg straight and the other slightly bent, ease your weight forwards towards the straight leg and feel the stretch at the back of the knee and thigh. Hold for 10 seconds, then change position and repeat with the other leg.

Chest Stretch Sitting with legs crossed or extended in front (whichever is more comfortable), raise your arms and clasp your hands behind your back to stretch the muscles across your chest. Hold for 10 seconds.

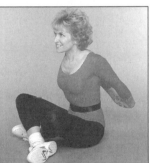

Upper Arm Stretch Sitting with legs crossed, ease one arm across the body, using the other arm to assist. Hold for 10 seconds. Relax, and repeat with the other arm.

Upper Back Stretch
Extend your arms forwards at shoulder level, rounding your back to separate your shoulder blades. Hold for 10 seconds.

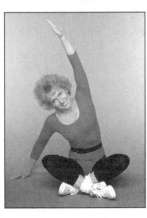

Waist Stretch Place one hand on the floor for support, and reach over to the side with the other arm. Hold for 10 seconds, then relax and repeat to the other side.

POSITIVE THOUGHT FOR THE DAY

You are over halfway through your first week of this Flat Stomach Plan. You must be feeling more confident, and now is the time to build on that. Confidence is created by a variety of conditions. We are conditioned by our environment, and if we mix with positive people we are likely to have a much more positive attitude. Our childhood experiences also affect our confidence, as do any previous experiences that we might have gone through. If we have a success experience it leads to a feeling of confidence which leads to a feeling of 'I can'. A failure experience leads to a feeling of 'I can't', or 'I'm no good at that' and a fear of failing. Our mind is an amazing storage area and, just as a computer can only put out information with which it has been programmed, it is the same with our mind. Whatever we put into our mind is what's going to come out of it. Appearance builds confidence possibly more than anything. Tomorrow put on your smartest outfit – one that also makes you look slimmer. Take extra trouble with your hair and make-up (if you are female!) and feel really good about how you are presenting yourself to the world. With this extra confidence you will find the whole day becomes a more pleasurable experience and you will find extra willpower to stick with the diet and the exercises. Look forward to tomorrow, don't cheat, and remember to maintain good posture at all times. Enjoy the feeling of being in control.

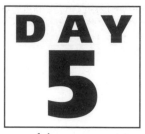

DAY 5

You are now well on the way to completing your first week of the programme. You should be feeling fitter, slimmer and much happier. Successful slimming is one of the most positive actions we can take to help us build confidence. People who do not have a weight problem or who do not mind being overweight have little understanding how those of us who *do* want to be slim can benefit from winning the battle. I would never persuade anyone to diet who didn't want to, but I know from personal experience how much better *I* feel if my weight is under control. When I discovered my *Hip and Thigh Diet*, which improved the shape of my body dramatically, my confidence factor rocketed and it enabled me to grow and embark on a career taking me in a number of directions and presenting me with challenges that I would never have believed I would be able to accomplish. Don't let anybody put you down or criticise your achievements. You are well on the way to achieving a wonderful new body. Think 'I *am* going to succeed, I *am* going to win'. Start spending more time on your appearance. The dividends it will pay will exceed all expectations. You will look better, you will *feel* better and you will command more respect from other people. It might take time, but it will work. Remember your posture, remember to smile, and enjoy your day. Realise that every time you go upstairs or every time you have to walk from one room to another you are helping your body to be fitter and leaner. Go for it!

MENU

BREAKFAST

1 oz (25 g) muesli mixed with 1 eating apple, peeled and coarsely grated, 1 small banana, chopped, 5 oz (125 g) low-fat natural yogurt, and 1 tsp honey or demerara sugar

or

1/4 pint/5 fl oz (125 ml) orange juice; 3/4 oz (18.5 g) porridge oats cooked with water and served with milk from allowance plus 1 tsp honey; 1 slice wholemeal toast spread with 1 tsp marmalade

LUNCH

ⓟ Roast Beef and Horseradish Sandwich

Spread 2 slices wholemeal bread with horseradish sauce. Fill with 2 oz (50 g) cold lean roast beef, and top with slices of radish and spring onion. Serve with salad

ⓠ 8 oz (200 g) jacket potato topped with 4 oz (100 g) baked beans and served with low-fat coleslaw and salad

ⓡ Trout and Spinach Salad (page 169)

DINNER

STARTER
Melon and Kiwi Salad

6 oz (150 g) water melon, chopped and mixed with 1 kiwi fruit, peeled and sliced

ⓡ Spaghetti Bolognese (page 161)

ⓠ Chicken Chop Suey (page 163)

ⓥ Vegetable Risotto (page 174)

DESSERT
Baked Banana (page 176)

WARM-UP

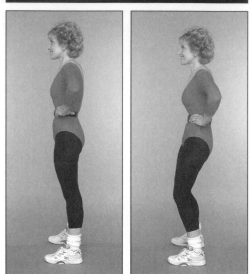

Stand in a good posture with your tummy in and your back straight, and tilt your pelvis forwards and upwards. Relax, and repeat. Do 8.

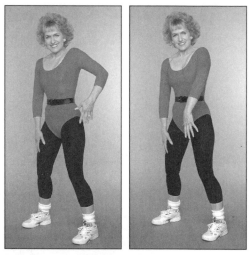

Roll alternate shoulders backwards, transferring your weight from one foot to the other. Do 16, then repeat, rolling shoulders forwards.

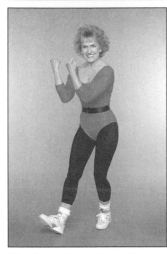

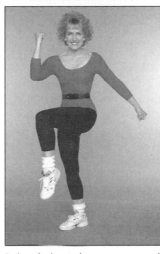

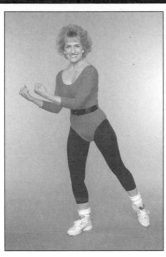

Step from side to side and tap the opposite heel on the floor in front, flexing and straightening your arms as you step. Do 16.

Take two steps to the side, making a scooping movement with your arms as if shovelling snow. Repeat to the other side. Do 16, alternating sides.

Raise alternate knees across and aim to touch with opposite elbow. Keep your tummy pulled in and your back straight. Do 16.

Take two steps to the side, swinging arms in and out as you step. Repeat to the other side. Do 16 to alternate sides.

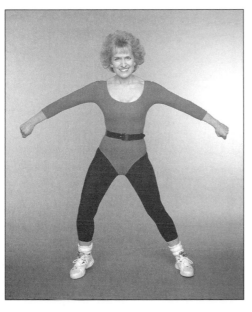

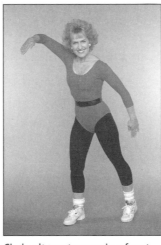

Circle alternate arms in a front crawl swimming motion, transferring your weight from one foot to the other. Do 16.

Back of Thigh Stretch
Bend one knee and, keeping your weight on that foot, extend the other leg in front, toes raised. Feel the stretch at the back of the knee and the thigh. Hold for 10 seconds, then change legs and repeat.

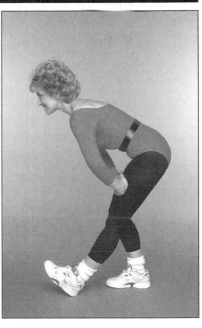

Calf Stretch Shift your weight on to the front leg and bend the knee. Your back leg is straight, heel on the floor and toes of both feet facing straight ahead. Keep your weight slightly forwards and feel the stretch in the calf muscle of your back leg. Hold for 10 seconds, then change legs and repeat.

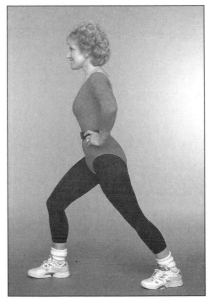

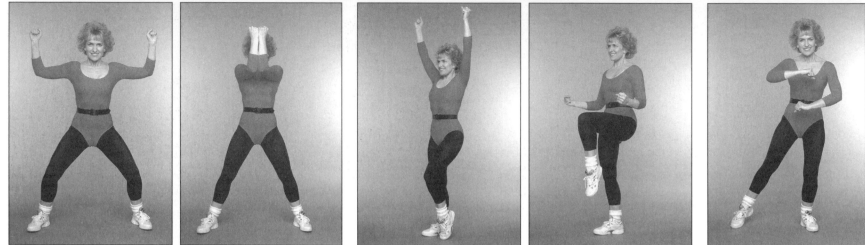

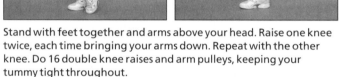

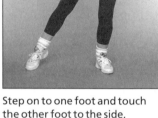

With feet wide apart and toes and knees facing slightly outwards, squat down, then come up again, bringing both arms out and in at shoulder level. Do 24.

Stand with feet together and arms above your head. Raise one knee twice, each time bringing your arms down. Repeat with the other knee. Do 16 double knee raises and arm pulleys, keeping your tummy tight throughout.

Step on to one foot and touch the other foot to the side, pressing down with alternate arms. Repeat to the other side. Do 16 to alternate sides.

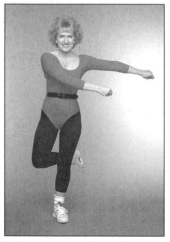

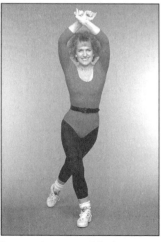

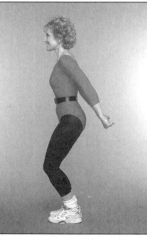

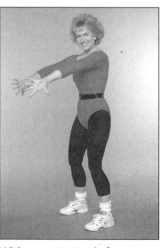

Swing your arms from side to side as you kick back with alternate feet. Do 32.

Step and curtsey with alternate legs, swinging your arms high and bringing them out and in to cross overhead. Do 24.

Alternately bend and straighten both knees, swinging your arms forwards and then pushing them back. Do 24.

With your arms out in front, rotate arms inwards and outwards 8 times.

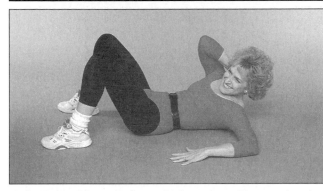 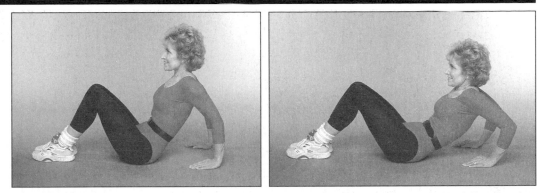

Waist Toner Lie on the floor with knees bent. Place one hand behind your head and have the other arm on the floor for support. Raise your head and shoulder and bring the elbow towards the opposite knee, taking care not to roll the hips. Return to the floor, and repeat. Do 12–14, then repeat to the other side.

Upper Arm Toner Sit with knees bent and prop yourself up on your hands. Your hands should be placed at least 12 inches (30 cm) behind your back, with fingers pointing forwards. Bend your arms so that your elbows move backwards, then straighten them again. Do 12–14.

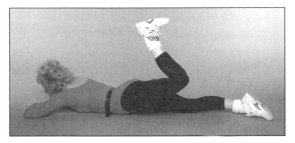 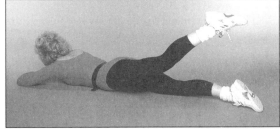 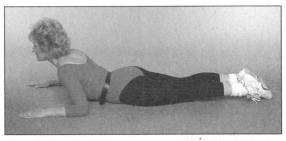

Back of Thigh Toner Lie face down and rest your head on your hands. Bend one leg and push the heel towards the ceiling, extending the leg slightly as you do so. Do 10–12, then repeat with the other leg.

Bottom Toner Still resting your head on your hands, raise one leg straight up and down, squeezing your seat as you raise. Keep your hips pressed into the floor throughout. Do 10–12, then repeat with the other leg.

Back Strengthener Lying with arms bent and palms down, slowly raise your chest and shoulders off the floor, using the muscles in your back not your arms. Return to the floor, and repeat. Do 8.

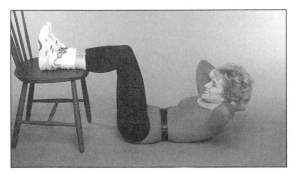

Tummy Toner Lie on your back with your feet placed against a wall or on a sturdy chair, and support your head with your hands. *Pulling your tummy in tightly*, raise your head and shoulders off the floor, keeping a distance between your chin and your chest. Raise on a count of 2, and return to the floor on a count of 2. Repeat 10–12 times.

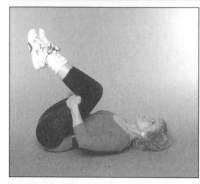

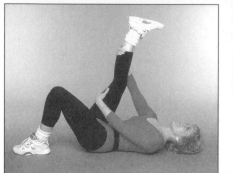

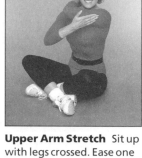

Seat Stretch Lie on your back with knees towards your chest and hold your hands underneath your thighs. Ease your legs further towards your chest and feel the stretch in your seat. Hold for 10 seconds.

Back of Thigh Stretch Lying with knees bent and feet flat on the floor, take hold of one leg and raise it, straightening it as far as is comfortable. Ease the leg towards you with your hands and hold for 10–15 seconds. Relax, and repeat with the other leg.

Upper Arm Stretch Sit up with legs crossed. Ease one arm across the body, using the other arm to assist. Hold for 10 seconds. Relax, and repeat with the other arm.

Tummy Stretch Lie face down with arms bent. Slowly raise your head and shoulders off the floor, supporting yourself on your forearms and elbows, and feel the stretch down the front of your abdomen. Hold for 10 seconds.

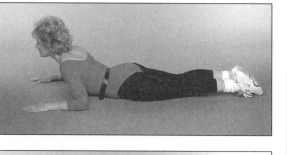

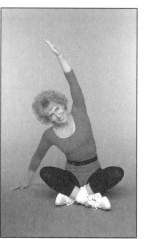

Back Stretch Position yourself on all fours and arch the spine as much as possible, pulling your tummy towards your spine. Hold for 10 seconds.

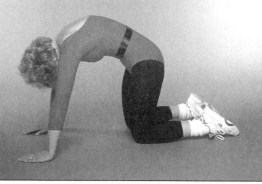

Waist Stretch Sitting with legs crossed, slowly reach over to the side with one arm, supporting yourself with the other arm. Hold for 10 seconds, then repeat to the other side.

POSITIVE THOUGHT FOR THE DAY

Yesterday we looked at the importance of building confidence and how our appearance can make a significant difference. When slimmers lose their excess pounds and are able to wear clothes that are several sizes smaller and look better, their confidence rockets. Because they feel so much more confident about the outside, the inside follows suit and they find themselves able to achieve things they never dared to attempt before. The *only* difference is confidence. Don't ever underestimate its value. Aim to strive towards it as each day goes by.

It is always good to build other people's confidence too. By so doing you demonstrate how confident *you* are. Telling someone how nice they look, how good they are at something or how kind they are makes that person feel better and enables them to 'grow'. Making positive comments about people is a valuable habit to develop. While we can't change experiences that might have forced us to lose confidence in the past, there is no reason why we shouldn't go forward and build confidence for the future. Sometimes people are reluctant to attempt a new challenge because of a fear of failure. Unless we aim for something worthwhile we are never likely to develop our character. Mix with people you admire. Watch how they behave and how they run their lives. Learn lessons from them. There is no point in re-inventing the wheel.

Continue to pay extra attention to your appearance as each day arrives. Enjoy your extra energy and your narrower waistline, and *feel* yourself succeeding on this programme. Life is going to get better and better from here on.

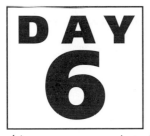

DAY 6

How are you feeling? You are nearly at the end of your first week so please continue to be saintly with the diet and as energetic as possible. Try on your skirt or trousers again today and see how much looser they are. Isn't it great when those inches start to disappear? Fat weighs little but it takes up a lot of space, and a low-fat diet will enable you to reduce the amount of fat on your body without your losing any of your muscle tissue. This is where crash diets are so harmful. Crash diets cause the body to use muscle tissue for energy, leaving the fat behind, and while people who follow crash diets may register a weight loss on the scales, in terms of body composition their level of fat will hardly have reduced. On the other hand, low-fat dieting is extremely effective in decreasing the amount of fat on the body, as are the exercises that we do each day. Realise that what you are doing is helping you not just for now but also for later years. It will help you towards better health, and give you greater energy and a fuller life.

Remember, if you need to do more or fewer repetitions of the aerobic or toning exercises you should adjust the number accordingly. In order to improve, it is necessary to 'challenge' the body. So do as many repetitions as is necessary to reach the point of fatigue but not pain.

Enjoy today's programme and look forward to the end of the week when it's weighing and measuring time. Do not get on the scales or use the tape measure yet. Use only the skirt or trousers as your progress guide. Enjoy your day.

MENU

BREAKFAST

8 oz (200 g) mixed berries plus ½ oz (12.5 g) Bran Flakes, topped with 5 oz (125 g) low-fat fromage frais or yogurt

or

1 slice (1½ oz/37.5 g) wholemeal toast with 2 tsp marmalade, plus 2 pieces fresh fruit

LUNCH

Ⓟ French Bread, Meat and Salad

2 oz (50 g) French bread spread with Branston pickle and topped with 2 oz (50 g) wafer-thin chicken or beef, plus salad
1 x 5 oz (125 g) diet yogurt

Ⓠ 1 x 16 oz (400 g) can Baxter's Cock-a-Leekie Soup plus 1 slice wholemeal toast (no butter); 1 piece fresh fruit and 1 x 5 oz (125 g) diet yogurt

Ⓡ Chinese Apple Salad
(page 160)

DINNER

STARTER
Melon and Prawn Salad
(page 157)

Ⓡ Chicken with Herby Lemon Sauce (page 163)

Ⓠ Beef Bourguignon (page 161)

Ⓥ Broccoli Delight (page 170)

DESSERT
Apple Meringue (page 175)

WARM-UP

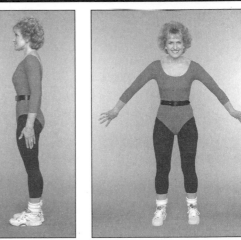

Start by standing tall, tummy in, shoulder blades back and down.

With your arms out to the sides, rotate arms forwards and backwards. Do 8

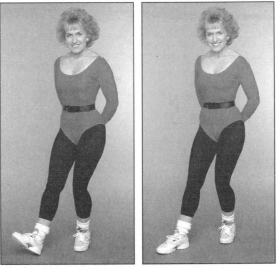

Raise the toes of one foot and tap the toes down to the floor 8 times. Repeat with the other foot.

CONTINUED ▶

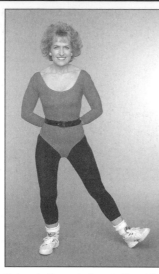

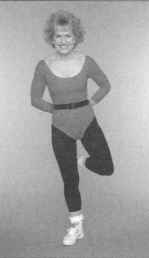

Tap alternate heels in front, flexing and straightening both arms. Do 16.

Extend alternate legs to the side, tapping the floor with your heels. Do 16.

Kick back with alternate feet. Do 16.

Back of Thigh Stretch

Bend one knee and, keeping your weight on that foot, extend the other leg in front, toes raised. Feel the stretch at the back of the knee and the thigh. Hold for 10 seconds, then change legs and repeat.

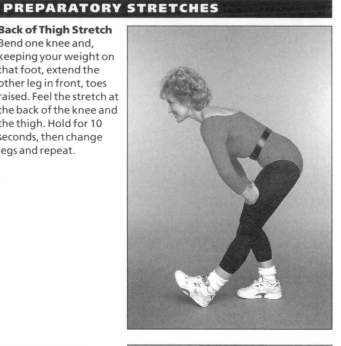

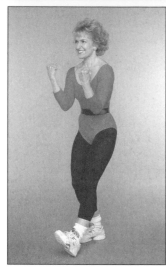

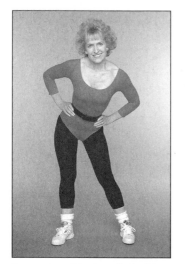

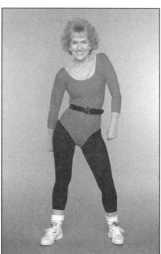

With feet a comfortable distance apart, raise one hip and at the same time raise the opposite shoulder. Repeat with the other hip and shoulder. Do 16 on alternate sides.

Rotate your hips in a clockwise direction. Do 8, then repeat in an anti-clockwise direction.

Calf Stretch Shift your weight on to the front leg and bend the knee. Your back leg is straight, heel on the floor and toes of both feet facing straight ahead. Keep your weight slightly forwards and feel the stretch in the calf muscle of your back leg. Hold for 10 seconds, then change legs and repeat.

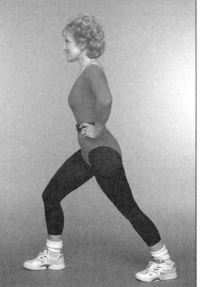

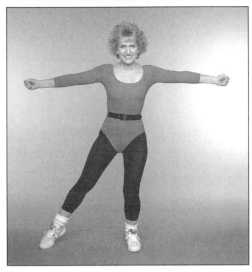

Extend alternate feet to the side, swinging the arms out and in at shoulder level. Do 16.

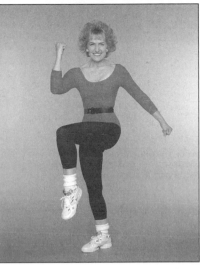

Raise alternate knees and aim to touch with opposite elbow. Keep the tummy tight. Do 32.

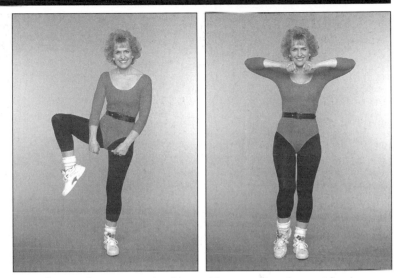

Raise alternate knees out to the side, pushing your arms down and up in 'barrow boy' style as you step. Do 24.

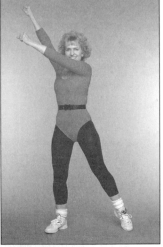

Step from side to side, swinging your arms high as you step. Do 24.

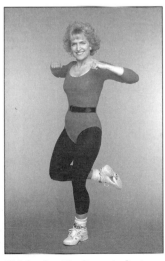

Kick back with alternate feet, bringing your arms backwards and forwards as you kick. Do 24.

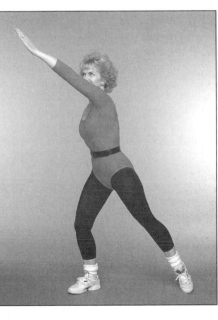

Step and lunge to one side, reaching across with the opposite arm. Straighten the arm and the opposite leg as much as possible so that only the toes of that foot touch the floor. Repeat to the other side. Do 24 to alternate sides.

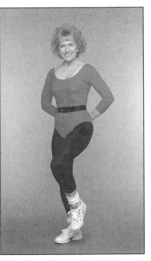

March on the spot with hands behind your back. Do 32 steps.

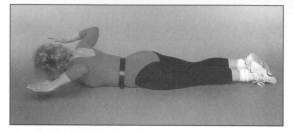

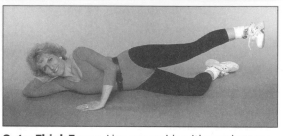

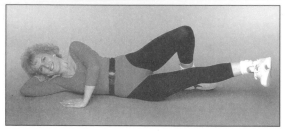

Upper Back Strengthener Lie face down with arms bent at shoulder level. Raise your arms, squeezing your shoulder blades together as much as possible. Lower your arms, and repeat. Do 10.

Outer Thigh Toner Lie on your side with your bottom leg bent and your top leg straight. Raise the top leg, keeping your hips square and your toes aiming slightly downwards. Do not raise the leg too high. Lower, then repeat. Do 12–14, then roll over and repeat with the other leg.

Inner Thigh Toner Bend the top leg and place the foot flat on the floor. Keeping the bottom leg straight, raise it as high as possible, making sure your hips remain square. Lower the leg, and repeat. Do 16, then roll over and repeat with the other leg.

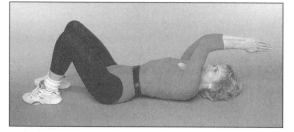

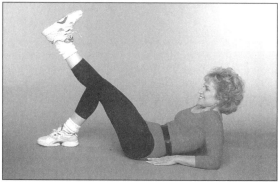

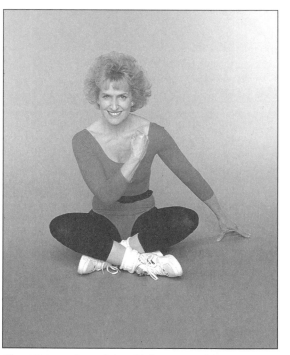

Chest Toner Lie on your back with knees bent and place your arms out to the sides with elbows bent at shoulder level. Lift your arms and press the elbows and palms together. Keeping the arms together and parallel with the floor, push them over your head and then pull them forwards again. Repeat this backwards and forwards movement 12–14 times, keeping the elbows together throughout the exercise.

Front Thigh Toner Support yourself on your elbows. One leg is bent and the other is extended on the floor. Raise the extended leg to the level of the bent leg, then lower it. Do 12–14, then repeat with the other leg.

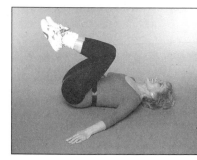

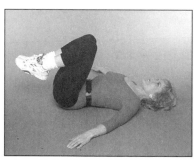

Tummy Trimmer Lie on your back with knees bent and raised, and pull your tummy in tightly. Pull your knees towards your chest while pressing down with your tummy muscles to lift the hips slightly off the floor. Do not use your arms to assist. Repeat 8–10 times.

Chest Toner Sit upright with legs crossed. Bend one elbow and press it against your chest as if holding a football to your chest and trying to squeeze the air out. Squeeze 12–14 times, then repeat with the other elbow.

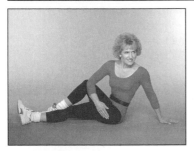

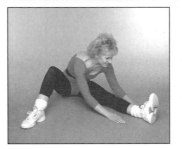

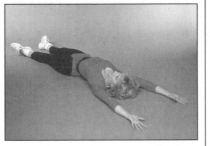

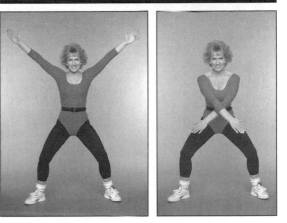

Waist and Outer Thigh Stretch Sit up straight with one leg extended and the other leg placed across it. Slowly twist your body away from the bent knee, using the opposite elbow to ease the bent knee further across. Hold for 10 seconds, then change legs and repeat to the other side.

Back of Thigh Stretch Sitting with one leg straight and the other slightly bent, ease your weight forwards towards the straight leg and feel the stretch at the back of the knee and the thigh. Hold for 10 seconds, then change the position of the legs to repeat on the other side.

Full Body Stretch Lie on your back and extend your arms and legs as much as possible. Hold for 10 seconds.

With feet wide apart, bend your knees and make sweeping circles with your arms. Do 24.

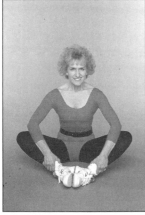

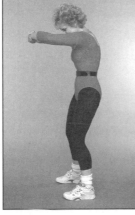

Inner Thigh Stretch Sit up with knees bent and soles of the feet together. Applying gentle pressure with your elbows, ease your knees outwards as far as is comfortable. Hold for 15 seconds.

Upper Back Stretch Stand with feet a comfortable distance apart and knees slightly bent. Round your back and raise your arms in front to shoulder level to separate your shoulder blades. Hold for 10 seconds.

Chest Stretch Stand with feet a comfortable distance apart and knees slightly bent. Take your arms behind you and place one hand on top of the other. Raise your arms to expand your chest. Feel the stretch across your chest. Hold for 10 seconds.

POSITIVE THOUGHT FOR THE DAY

We all have good days and bad days and anyone who has ambition is bound to have days when they lack confidence. If you don't, then you don't have any goals. No one ever goes through life on a straight rosy path without any problems or difficulties. Life just isn't like that. If you find that during your diet and fitness programme one day you do cheat a little, don't get so disheartened that you throw in the towel. Instead, pick yourself up and acknowledge that, whatever the indiscretion might have been, it will not cause a huge amount of damage. Providing you go straight back on to the diet as described, you will be able to repair that damage very quickly. So often it is not that one chocolate biscuit that does the damage. It's eating the whole packet. If you *have* to cheat, keep it to an absolute minimum and then forget about it. Try and be more physically active to compensate, and try to lengthen the gap in the days between each 'cheat'. Soon you will build your confidence so that *you* are in control of the 'cheats', rather than letting them control you. You will be so confident in your ability to control your food intake that these problems will be something of the past.

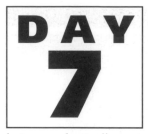

DAY 7

Here you are on Day 7. Brilliant! You are nearly at the end of your first week. Well done! Today, concentrate on your posture and on being as physically active as possible. Look upon it as a day of achievement and activity. You are going to weigh and measure yourself tomorrow, so today's the day to call on every ounce of enthusiasm and willpower to enable you to stick to the diet and execute the exercises with extra zeal. It's the day you're not even going to think about cheating and the day to smile at your own achievement of getting to the end of your first week. The 'measuring' skirt or pair of trousers is getting looser. You are feeling good about yourself and you're coping with the diet and the exercises, fitting them into your daily schedule, feeling an enormous sense of achievement having done them and already seeing results. Really enjoy today and look forward to tomorrow morning. Whatever you do, don't waver or even consider having anything extra to eat. If you feel the slightest inclination, pour yourself a low-calorie diet drink, then go outside and do some physical activity. Really go for it today.

MENU

BREAKFAST

8 oz (200 g) tinned grapefruit in natural juice

or

1 whole grapefruit; 1 oz (25 g) grilled lean bacon, plus 1 egg, dry-fried in a non-stick pan, and 1 slice light bread, toasted

LUNCH

Ⓟ Cottage Cheese and Pineapple Roll

Finely slice a spring onion and mix with 1 heaped tbsp low-fat cottage cheese. Add some chopped pineapple (canned in natural juice) and a few slices of orange. Spread a crusty roll or French stick (2 oz/50 g) with reduced-oil salad dressing and add the cottage cheese filling

Ⓠ 2 slices wholemeal toast topped with 1 x 8 oz (200 g) can spaghetti in tomato sauce; 1 piece fresh fruit

Ⓡ Smoked Mackerel or Salmon Salad

4 oz (100 g) smoked mackerel or salmon with large mixed salad, 1 tsp horseradish sauce and 1 tsp oil-free salad dressing
1 piece fresh fruit and 1 x 5 oz (125 g) diet yogurt

DINNER

STARTER
Orange and Grapefruit Cocktail
(page 157)

Ⓡ **Roast Chicken and Potato and Parsley Bake** (page 175)

Ⓠ **Coq au Vin** (page 165)

Ⓥ **Vegetable and Herb Bake** (page 174)

DESSERT
Baked Stuffed Apple (page 176)

WARM-UP

Start by checking your posture. Stand tall with tummy in and shoulder blades back and down.

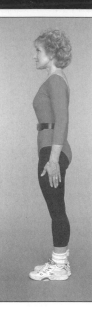

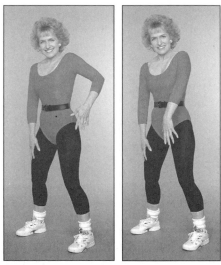

Roll alternate shoulders backwards, transferring your weight from one foot to the other. Do 16, then repeat, rolling shoulders forwards.

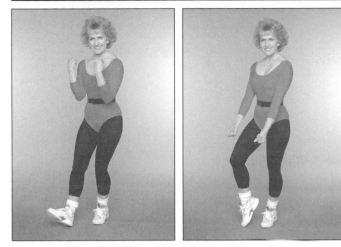

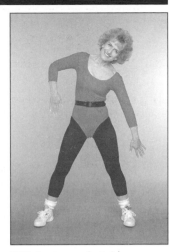

Tap the heel and then the toe of one foot, flexing and straightening both arms. Do 8, then repeat with the other foot.

With feet a comfortable distance apart, lean over to the side without twisting the hips. Repeat to the other side. Do 8 to each side.

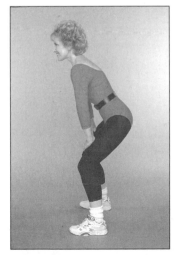

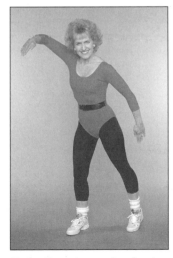

With feet wide apart, bend your knees and squat down. Make sure your knees bend over the ankles. Come up again, and repeat. Do 8.

Circle alternate arms in a front crawl swimming motion, transferring your weight from one foot to the other. Do 16.

Back of Thigh Stretch
Bend one knee and, keeping your weight on that foot, extend the other leg in front, toes raised. Feel the stretch at the back of the knee and the thigh. Hold for 10 seconds, then change legs and repeat.

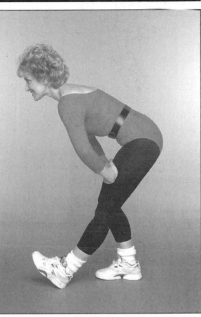

Calf Stretch Shift your weight on to the front leg and bend the knee. Your back leg is straight, heel on the floor and toes of both feet facing straight ahead. Keep your weight slightly forwards and feel the stretch in the calf muscle of your back leg. Hold for 10 seconds, then change legs and repeat.

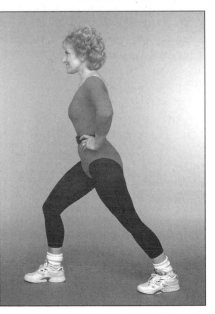

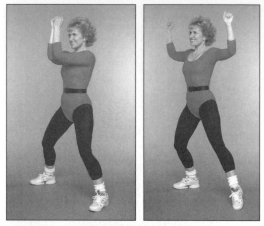
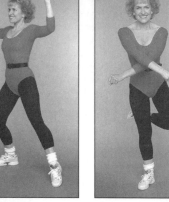
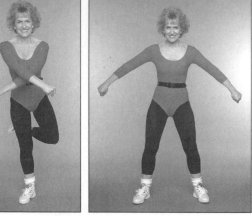

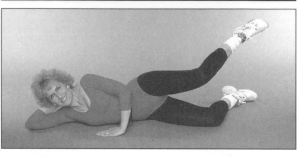

With feet wide apart, transfer your weight from one foot to the other, opening and closing your bent arms at shoulder level.

Kick back with alternate feet, swinging arms out and in to cross in front. Do 24.

Outer Thigh Toner Lie on your side and bend both knees. Raise and then lower the top leg, keeping it bent. Make sure the hips are square and the knees and toes face forwards. Do 12–14, then roll over, and repeat with the other leg.

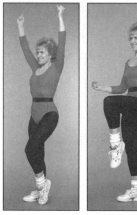
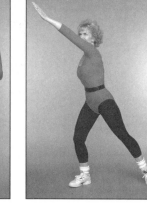
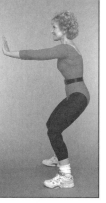

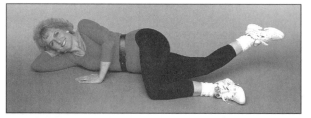

Inner Thigh Toner Keep the top leg bent and rest it on the floor in front of you. Raise the bottom leg, keeping it slightly bent. Lower the leg, and repeat. Do 12–14, then roll over and repeat with the other leg.

Stand with feet together and arms above your head. Raise one knee twice, each time bringing your arms down. Repeat with the other knee. Do 16 double knee raises and arm pulleys, keeping your tummy tight throughout.

Step and lunge to one side, reaching across with the opposite arm. Straighten the arm and the opposite leg as much as possible so that only the toes of that foot touch the floor. Repeat to the other side. Do 24 to alternate sides.

With feet wide apart and knees and toes facing slightly outwards, bend the knees into a squatting position, pushing your hands forwards as you squat. Raise, and repeat. Do 10.

Do a walking jog on the spot, punching alternate hands forwards as you step. Do 30.

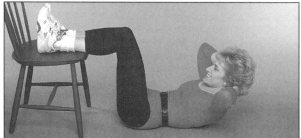

Tummy Toner Lie on your back with your feet placed against a wall or on a sturdy chair, and support your head with your hands. *Pulling your tummy in tightly*, raise your head and shoulders off the floor, keeping a distance between your chin and your chest. Raise on a count of 2, and return to the floor on a count of 2. Repeat 12–14 times.

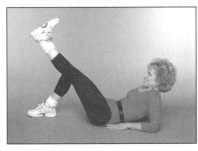

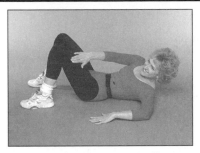

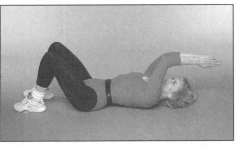

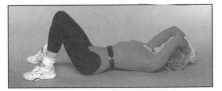

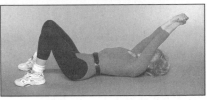

Front Thigh Toner Support yourself on your elbows. One leg is bent and the other is extended on the floor. Raise the extended leg to the level of the bent leg, then lower it. Do 12–14, then repeat with the other leg.

Waist Toner Lie back on the floor. Supporting yourself with one arm, reach across your body with the other arm, pressing your tummy down as you reach. Take care not to roll the hips. Return to the floor, and repeat. Do 8–10, then repeat to the other side.

Chest Toner Still lying on the floor with knees bent, place your arms out to the sides with elbows bent at shoulder level. Lift your arms and press the elbows and palms together. Keeping the arms together and parallel with the floor, push them over your head and then pull them forwards again. Repeat this backwards and forwards movement 12–14 times, keeping the elbows together throughout the exercise.

Upper Arm Toner Bend your arms and place them over your head. Straighten your arms, then bend them again. Repeat this movement 12–14 times.

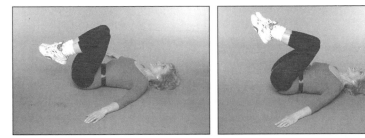

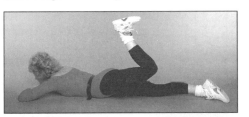

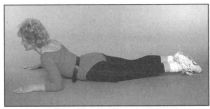

Tummy Trimmer Lying on your back with knees bent and raised, pull your tummy in tightly. Pull your knees towards your chest while pressing down with your tummy muscles to lift the hips slightly off the floor. Do not use your arms to assist. Repeat 12–14 times.

Back of Thigh Toner Lie on your front and rest your head on your hands. Bend one leg and push the heel towards the ceiling, extending the leg slightly as you do so. Do 10–12, then repeat with the other leg.

Back Strengthener Lying with arms bent and palms down, slowly raise your chest and shoulders off the floor, using the muscles in your back not your arms. Return to the floor, and repeat. Do 8–10.

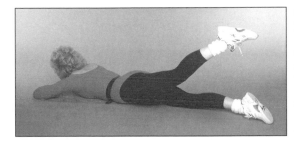

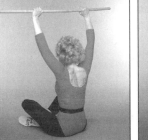

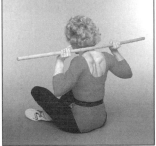

Bottom Toner Rest your head on your hands. Raise one leg straight up and down, squeezing your seat as you raise. Keep your hips pressed into the floor throughout. Do 10–12, then repeat with the other leg.

Shoulder Strengthener Take a pole and sit upright in a comfortable position. Raise the pole above your head, then lower it, squeezing your shoulder blades together. Repeat. Do 12–14, concentrating on bringing your shoulder blades together as you lower the pole.

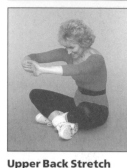

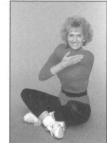

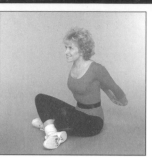

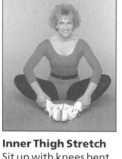

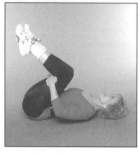

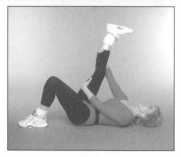

Upper Back Stretch
Sitting with legs crossed, round your back and raise your arms in front to shoulder level to separate your shoulder blades. Hold for 10 seconds.

Chest Stretch Keeping your legs crossed or extending them in front (whichever is more comfortable), raise your arms and clasp your hands behind your back to stretch the muscles across your chest. Hold for 10 seconds.

Upper Arm Stretch Ease one arm across the body, using the other arm to assist. Hold for 10 seconds. Relax, and repeat with the other arm.

Inner Thigh Stretch Sit up with knees bent and soles of the feet together. Using your elbows, gently ease your knees down as far as is comfortable. Hold for 15 seconds.

Seat Stretch Lie on your back with knees towards your chest and place your hands underneath your thighs. Ease your legs further towards your chest and feel the stretch in your seat. Hold for 10 seconds.

Back of Thigh Stretch Lie on your back with knees bent. Take hold of one leg and raise it, straightening it as far as is comfortable. Ease the leg towards you with your hands and hold for 10–15 seconds. Relax, and repeat with the other leg.

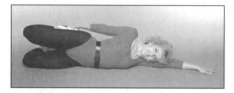

Front Thigh Stretch Lie on your side with both legs bent. Keeping the hips square, ease the foot of the top leg back, using your hand to assist. Hold for 10 seconds. Roll over and repeat with the other leg.

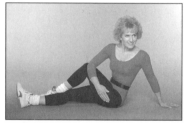

Waist and Outer Thigh Stretch
Sit up straight with one leg extended and the other leg placed across it. Slowly twist your body away from the bent knee, using the opposite elbow to ease the bent knee further across. Hold for 10 seconds, then change legs and repeat to the other side.

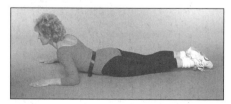

Tummy Stretch Lie face down with arms bent. Slowly raise your head and shoulders off the floor, supporting yourself on your forearms and elbows, and feel the stretch down the front of your abdomen. Hold for 10 seconds.

POSITIVE THOUGHT FOR THE DAY

It is very important to remember that when we are following a diet and fitness programme persistence is crucial. Failure cannot live with persistence, and if you persevere and stick to the diet and do the exercises, in the end I promise you will succeed. Remember that we cannot fail at anything until we actually give up. Even if you have never succeeded on a diet or an exercise programme before, let *this* be your first success experience. Remember, it isn't diets or exercise programmes that fail, it is those who follow them that fail through lack of perseverance. Great inventors didn't just hit upon their incredible discoveries by accident one day. They worked on them for months and years in some cases in order to develop the ultimate answer. The same principle applies with this diet and exercise programme. If you stick with it and really work at it you will reap the rewards, not just in the short but also in the long term.

Life can be so good, and those of us that are privileged enough to enjoy good health should be able to live it to the absolute maximum. No matter how old we are, we can all benefit from exercise. The benefits are very real and remarkably quick too, which is very encouraging. If we exercise for a couple of weeks we will certainly begin to see the improvement in both our energy levels and our body shape. Start picturing yourself succeeding and don't have any fear of failure. Give yourself a great big pat on the back because you have now finished the first week. Brilliant! Don't stop now.

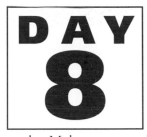
Well, this is it, the day you have been working towards for the last week. It's time to weigh and measure yourself to see how much progress you have made. Make sure you go to the bathroom before you weigh yourself. Place your scales on a flat board and weigh yourself in exactly the same clothes – or no clothes – that you wore when you weighed in on Day 1. Note your new weight in the appropriate box on the Weight and Inch Loss Record Chart. Now measure yourself carefully. Note down each measurement and tot up the total inches you have lost during this first week. Now you can see that all your hard work, effort and self-discipline really has paid dividends. Take a good look at yourself in the mirror and see how much your shape has improved during this first week. You are now 25 per cent of the way towards your first major goal. You should be thrilled by your progress, and you should now feel and see a real difference in the clothes you wear. Look forward to the next week, perform the exercises with lots of energy. *Be as physically active as you can every day* and don't cheat by eating in between meals. If there was a menu last week that you particularly enjoyed, feel free to go back and repeat it. This diet is designed to fit in with your lifestyle, your tastes and your purse. If you can make it work for you, you will succeed. Remember, aerobic exercise – that's exercise that makes us puff a bit and makes the heart beat faster – burns fat. Be as physically active as you can and see your energy levels grow and grow. Put on a smile, stand tall, and enjoy your day.

MENU

BREAKFAST

1/4 pint/5 fl oz (125 ml) orange juice; 2 slices light bread, toasted, or 1 medium slice (1 1/2 oz/37.5 g) wholemeal toast, topped with 1 x 8 oz (200 g) can baked beans

or

12 oz (300 g) fresh fruit, chopped and mixed with 10 oz (250 g) diet yogurt

LUNCH

P Chicken and Salad Sandwich
2 slices wholemeal bread spread with reduced-oil salad dressing and filled with 2 oz (50 g) ham or chicken, plus salad
1 piece fresh fruit

Q 1 Batchelor's Slim a Soup, plus 1 slice light wholemeal bread (no butter); 2 pieces fresh fruit and 1 Shape Twinpot yogurt

R Fruit and Chicken Salad (page 160)

DINNER

STARTER
Melon Balls in Slimline Ginger Ale
Use 6 oz (150 g) melon and scoop out flesh with a ball-scoop. Pour ginger ale over.

R Baked Haddock (page 167)

O Chinese Menu 1 (page 162)
Beef in Black Bean Sauce, Sweet and Sour Pork, Chicken in Spicy Tomato Sauce

V Vegetable Chilli (page 173)

DESSERT
1 Meringue Biscuit (page 178) or meringue nest filled with 4 oz (100 g) fresh fruit of your choice topped with 2 oz (50 g) low-fat yogurt or fromage frais

WARM-UP

With your arms behind your back, rotate arms inwards and outwards. Do 8.

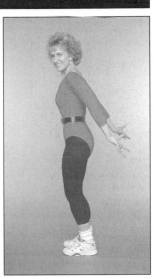

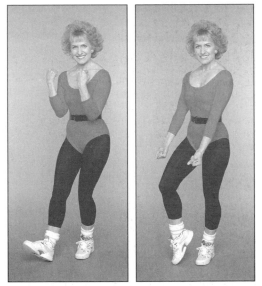

Tap the heel and then the toe of one foot, flexing and straightening both arms. Do 8, then repeat with the other foot.

CONTINUED ▶

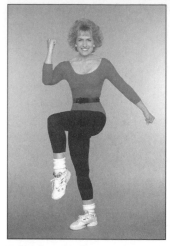

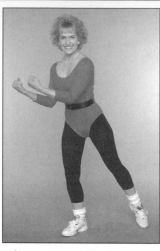

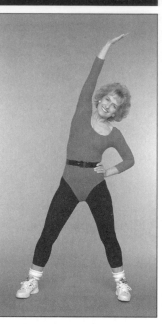

Back of Thigh Stretch
Bend one knee and, keeping your weight on that foot, extend the other leg in front, toes raised. Feel the stretch at the back of the knee and the thigh. Hold for 10 seconds, then change legs and repeat.

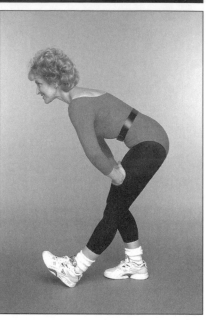

Raise alternate knees across and aim to touch with opposite elbow. Keep your tummy pulled in and your back straight. Do 16.

Take two steps to the side, making a scooping movement with your arms as if shovelling snow. Repeat to the other side. Do 16, alternating sides.

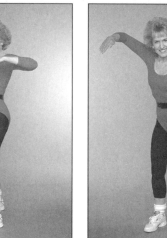

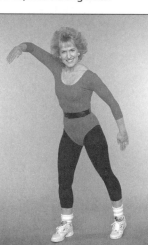

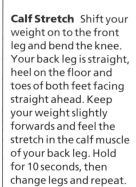

Stand with feet a comfortable distance apart, one arm raised with palm facing upwards, the other hand on your hip. Lean directly to the side, reaching over with the raised arm. Do not twist the hips. Return to the starting position and repeat to the other side. Do 8 to each side.

Calf Stretch Shift your weight on to the front leg and bend the knee. Your back leg is straight, heel on the floor and toes of both feet facing straight ahead. Keep your weight slightly forwards and feel the stretch in the calf muscle of your back leg. Hold for 10 seconds, then change legs and repeat.

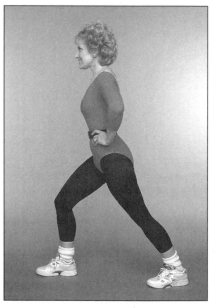

Keeping your hips square, twist your upper body from side to side. Do not jerk. Do 8 to each side

Circle alternate arms in a front crawl swimming motion, transferring your weight from one foot to the other. Do 16.

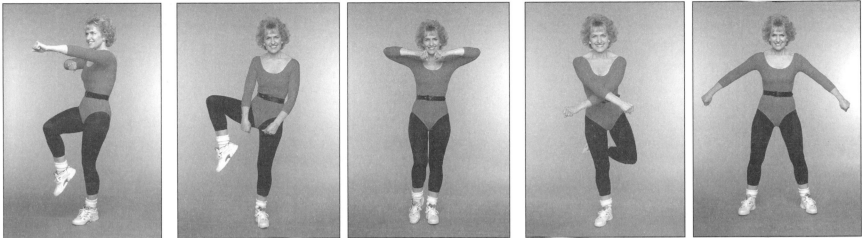

March on the spot, punching alternate hands forwards. Don't stamp. Do 24.

Raise alternate knees out to the side, pushing your arms down and up in 'barrow boy' style as you step. Do 24.

Kick back with alternate feet, swinging your arms out and in and crossing them in front. Do 24.

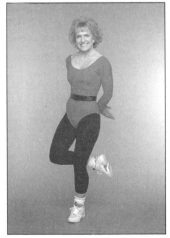
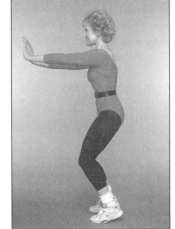
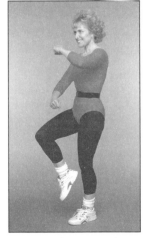
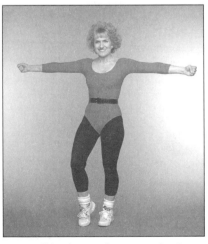
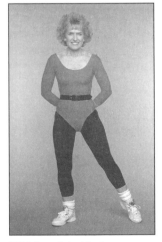

Continue to kick back with alternate feet, swinging your arms out and in and crossing them behind. Do 24.

With knees close together, dip down, bending the knees, then come up again, swinging your arms forwards and backwards. Do 32.

March on the spot and beat an imaginary drum with your hands. Do 32.

Do a walking jog on the spot and swing your arms in and out at shoulder level, bending then straightening them. Do 24.

With hands behind your back, step from side to side, transferring your weight from one foot to the other as you step. Do 24.

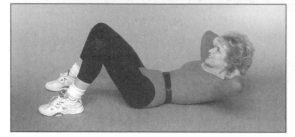

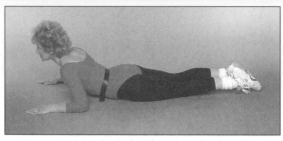

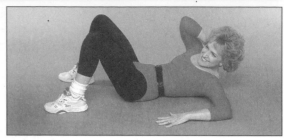

Tummy Toner Lie on your back with knees bent and your *tummy pulled in tightly*. Place your hands behind your neck and slowly raise your head and shoulders off the floor. Raise on a count of 2, then return to the floor on a count of 2, keeping a distance between your chin and your chest. Breathe out as you raise and breathe in as you go down. Do 6–10.

Back Strengthener Lie face down with arms bent, shoulder level, palms facing upwards. Slowly raise your chest off the floor, using the muscles in your back not your arms. Return to the floor and repeat. Do 8–10.

Waist Toner Lie on your back with knees bent. Place one hand behind your neck and have the other arm on the floor for support. Raise the head and shoulder and bring your elbow towards the opposite knee, taking care not to roll your hips. Return to the floor, and repeat. Do 12–14, then repeat to the other side.

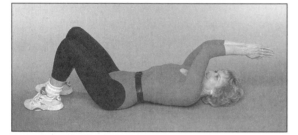

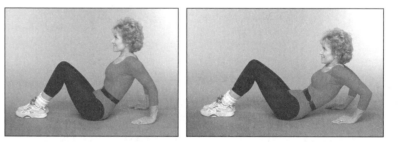

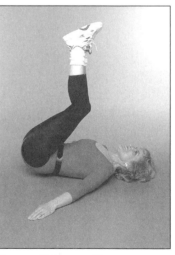

Chest Toner Still lying on the floor with knees bent, place your arms out to the sides with elbows bent at shoulder level. Lift your arms and press the elbows and palms together. Keeping the arms together and parallel with the floor, push them over your head and then pull them forwards again. Repeat this backwards and forwards movement 10–12 times, keeping the elbows together throughout the exercise.

Upper Arm Toner Sit with knees bent and prop yourself up on your hands. Your hands should be placed at least 12 inches (30 cm) behind your back, with fingers pointing forwards. Bend your arms so that your elbows move backwards, then straighten them again. Do 10–12.

Tummy Trimmer Lie on your back with legs raised and slightly bent. Your feet are over your hips and your tummy is pulled in tightly. Press your tummy muscles down and lift the hips slightly off the floor. Repeat 10–12 times, ensuring the effort comes from your abdomen, not your arms.

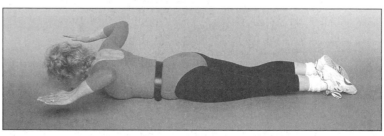

Upper Back Strengthener Lie face down with arms bent at shoulder level. Raise your arms, squeezing your shoulder blades together as much as possible, then lower your arms. Repeat 12–14 times.

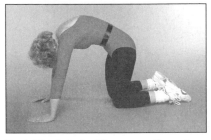

Back Stretch Position yourself on all fours and arch the spine as much as possible, pulling your tummy towards your spine. Hold for 10 seconds.

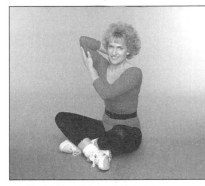

Back of Upper Arm Stretch Raise one elbow and ease your hand down your back. Use the other arm to ease it further. Hold for 10 seconds. Repeat with the other arm.

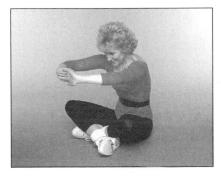

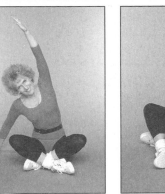

Waist Stretch Sit up with legs crossed. Place one hand on the floor for support, and reach over to the side with the other arm. Hold for 10 seconds, then relax and repeat to the other side.

Chest Stretch Keeping your legs crossed or extending them in front (whichever is more comfortable), raise your arms and clasp your hands behind your back to stretch the muscles across your chest. Hold for 10 seconds.

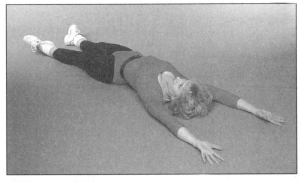

Full Body Stretch Lie on your back and extend your arms and legs as much as possible. Hold for 10 seconds.

Upper Back Stretch Sitting with legs crossed, reach your arms forwards, and round your back to separate the shoulder blades. Keep the arms at shoulder level. Hold for 10 seconds.

POSITIVE THOUGHT FOR THE DAY

Having weighed and measured yourself this morning you must be very pleased with the results that you have already achieved. This will spur you on for the next seven days and to your next weigh in. Go forward with confidence and determination, and you can't fail.

This week I would like us to look at how we can improve the quality of our life by looking at what we do both at home and in our work and to see how we can do it better. As soon as we start developing a positive outlook our attitude to everything around us becomes more positive and constructive. Make a list of the jobs that you presently have to do which you really loathe. Similarly, make a list of all the jobs and tasks and hobbies that you enjoy doing and try to develop a plan within your weekly schedule to enable you to do more of the things that you enjoy and less of the things that you do not. At work there may be jobs that you really do not like doing. Is there any way that these could be delegated or that you could receive some help with them? Are there any chores at home which you might be able to delegate to another member of the family? Mothers tend to be martyrs and try to do everything themselves, feeling, unwisely, that if they don't do everything themselves either it isn't going to be done properly or they haven't fulfilled their proper role as a mother. This is nonsense of course. Asking the whole family to join in and help not only helps to educate children in learning useful tasks for later life, but it also creates a feeling of teamwork within the family. At the risk of becoming very unpopular with your family (!) I suggest that you start making a list of which jobs could be done and by whom. Perhaps they could all be done at the same time so that everyone is busy doing their chores together. As a 'reward' the whole family could then go out and participate in some physical activity, such as swimming or walking. We can all fit so much more into our lives if we are well organised. We waste a great deal of our lives through bad planning or not planning at all. Start thinking about how you can improve the 'quality' time that you spend with your family. Delegation is not a dirty word!

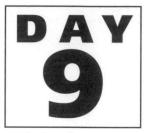

DAY 9

Try on your skirt or trousers again today and see the difference compared with just over a week ago. Never ever part with this item of clothing. Keep it as a constant reminder of your progress.

For a diet to be successful in the long term it is important to make some changes in your day-to-day life. The food that made you overweight in the first place and the lack of activity that caused you to be unfit and lethargic have to be considered as part of your past. From now on, your activity level is going to increase and the dietary changes you have made will become part of your new way of life. If you maintain these new lifestyle changes you will never regain your lost weight. Eat in moderation, and try to put maximum energy into every physical activity you do throughout the day. Just *being* more active will enable you to increase your fitness level, but think how you could improve your fitness even *more* if you took up exercise on a regular basis and combined it with an increased level of activity in your everyday life. The improvements would be far greater and will happen much more quickly.

Today's exercises are more challenging and will benefit your body even more now that it is accustomed to using a variety of muscles that may have done little work in recent years. Each day you are using different sets of muscles in an attempt to give your body an all-round workout. Realise which muscles are working. Feel them getting stronger. Enjoy today's menus and eat sufficient with your evening meal so that you don't feel the inclination to nibble later. Enjoy your day.

MENU

BREAKFAST

¼ pint/5 fl oz (125 ml) orange juice; 2 oz (50 g) any cereal with milk from allowance plus 1 tsp demerara sugar

or

¼ pint/5 fl oz (125 ml) orange juice; wholemeal bread roll (1½ oz/37.5 g) spread with mustard and filled with 2 oz (50 g) wafer-thin ham

LUNCH

P 2 slices wholemeal bread spread with 2 tsp horseradish sauce topped with sliced beetroot and sweetcorn; 1 x 8 oz (200 g) pot Müllerlight yogurt

Q 1 x 16 oz (400 g) can Baxter's Mediterranean Tomato Soup with Selected Vegetables, plus 1 slice wholemeal toast (no butter) 1 x 5 oz (125 g) diet yogurt

R *Cottage Cheese, Coleslaw and Bean Sprout Pitta*

1 wholemeal pitta filled with 2 oz (50 g) low-fat cottage cheese, low-fat coleslaw, bean sprouts, shredded lettuce, sliced tomato, cucumber, onion and pepper
1 x 5 oz (125 g) diet yogurt

DINNER

STARTER
Mixed Salad with Garlic and Yogurt Dressing
(page 179)

R *Tarragon Chicken* (page 166)

Q Findus Lean Cuisine Prawn Curry with Rice

V *Blackeye Bean Casserole* (page 169)

DESSERT
4 oz (100 g) frozen yogurt (any brand)

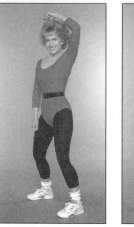

Rotate alternate arms backwards as if brushing your hair, transferring your weight from one foot to the other. Do 16.

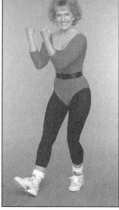

Step from side to side and tap the opposite heel on the floor in front, flexing and straightening your arms as you step. Do 16.

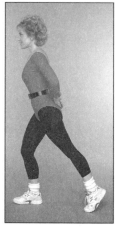

Tap alternate feet on the floor behind you. Do 32.

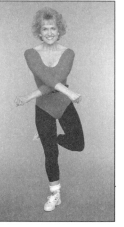

Kick back with alternate feet, crossing your arms in front. Do 16.

WARM-UP

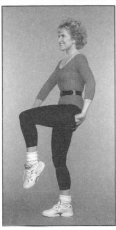

Raise alternate knees in front, pressing down with both arms. Keep your tummy tight and back straight. Do 16.

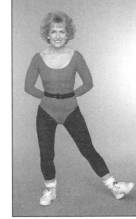

Extend alternate legs to the side, tapping the floor with your heels. Do 16.

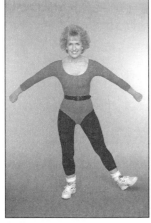

Extend alternate legs to the side, tapping the floor with your heels and swinging your arms in and out. Do 16.

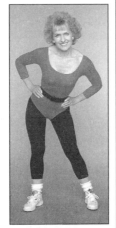

Rotate your hips in a clockwise direction. Do 8, then repeat in an anti-clockwise direction.

PREPARATORY STRETCHES

Back of Thigh Stretch Bend one knee and, keeping your weight on that foot, extend the other leg in front, toes raised. Feel the stretch at the back of the knee and the thigh. Hold for 10 seconds, then change legs and repeat.

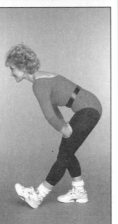

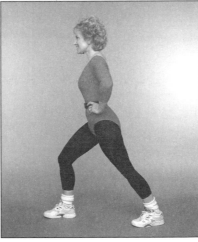

Calf Stretch Shift your weight on to the front leg and bend the knee. Your back leg is straight, heel on the floor and toes of both feet facing straight ahead. Keep your weight slightly forwards and feel the stretch in the calf muscle of your back leg. Hold for 10 seconds, then change legs and repeat.

AEROBIC

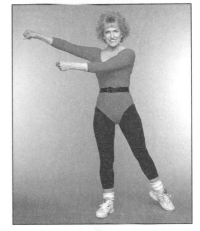

Alternately bend and straighten your knees, pulling your elbows back at shoulder level and keeping your tummy pulled in tightly. Do 32.

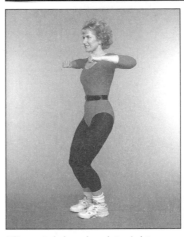

Extend alternate legs to the side, pointing your toes and swinging your arms from side to side. Do 32.

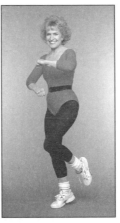

Jog on the spot, pressing down with alternate arms. Make sure your knees are soft and your heels are down when you land. Do 32.

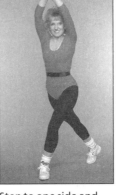

Step to one side and curtsey, swinging your arms out and in to cross high above your head. Do 24.

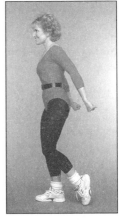

Tap the toes of one foot on the floor behind, pushing your arms back as you step. Do 32 with alternate feet.

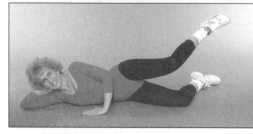

Outer Thigh Toner Lie on your side and bend both knees. Raise and then lower the top leg, keeping it bent. Make sure the hips are square and the knees and toes face forwards. Do 12–14, then roll over, and repeat with the other leg.

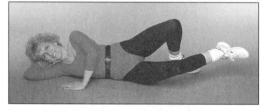

Inner Thigh Toner Place the foot of the top leg flat on the floor behind the bent lower leg. Raise the bottom leg as high as possible, keeping it slightly bent and making sure your hips remain square. Lower the leg, and repeat. Do 12–14, then roll over, and repeat with the other leg.

Bottom Toner
Face the chair and raise one leg behind you, keeping the leg straight and squeezing your seat as you raise. Lower the leg, and repeat. Keep your tummy tight, hips square and your back straight throughout. Do 12–14, then repeat with the other leg.

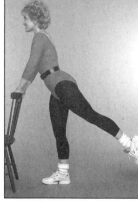

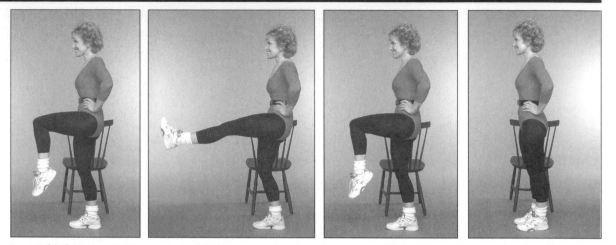

Front Thigh Toner Holding on to a chair for support, bend one knee, extend it straight out in front, then bend it again and return to the starting position. Keep your tummy in and your back straight throughout. Repeat this sequence 10–12 times, then turn round and repeat with the other leg.

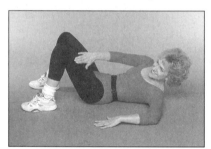

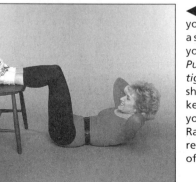

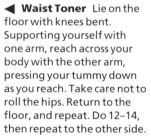

◄ **Waist Toner** Lie on the floor with knees bent. Supporting yourself with one arm, reach across your body with the other arm, pressing your tummy down as you reach. Take care not to roll the hips. Return to the floor, and repeat. Do 12–14, then repeat to the other side.

◄ **Tummy Toner** Place your feet against a wall or on a sturdy chair, and support your head with your hands. *Pulling your tummy in tightly*, raise your head and shoulders off the floor, keeping a distance between your chin and your chest. Raise on a count of 2, and return to the floor on a count of 2. Repeat 12–14 times.

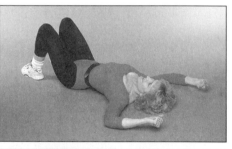

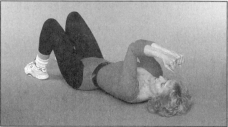

▲ **Chest Toner** Place your arms out to the sides, elbows bent and level with your shoulders. Lift your arms and press the elbows together. Lower the arms, and repeat. Do 12–14.

TONING

Inner Thigh Toner

Lying on your back with arms outstretched and knees bent and raised above your hips, separate your knees and then bring them together again, keeping your back pressed into the floor. Do 12–14.

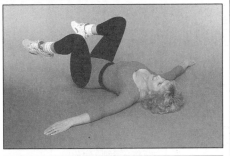

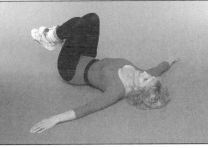

Tummy Trimmer

Still lying on your back with knees bent and raised, pull your tummy in tightly. Pull your knees towards your chest while pressing down with your tummy muscles to lift the hips slightly off the floor. Do not use your arms to assist. Repeat 12–14 times.

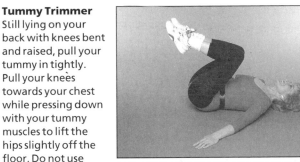

COOL-DOWN STRETCHES

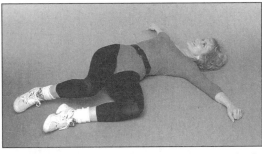

Outer Thigh Stretch Lying with arms outstretched and knees bent, lower both knees slowly to one side, keeping both feet on the floor. Hold for 10 seconds. Slowly raise the knees to the centre, and repeat to the other side.

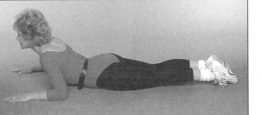

Tummy Stretch Lie face down with arms bent. Slowly raise your head and shoulders off the floor, supporting yourself on your forearms and elbows, and feel the stretch down the front of your abdomen. Hold for 10 seconds.

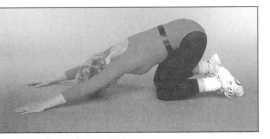

Seat Stretch Start in the all fours position. Slowly ease your hips backwards without touching your heels and, at the same time, extend your arms in front. Hold for 10 seconds

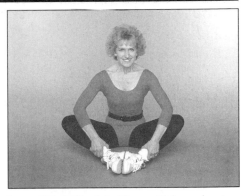

Inner Thigh Stretch Sit up with knees bent and soles of the feet together. Using your elbows, gently ease your knees down as far as is comfortable. Hold for 15 seconds

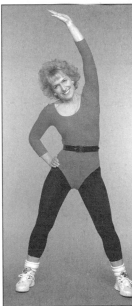

Waist Stretch Standing with feet a comfortable distance apart and knees slightly bent, place one hand on your thigh for support and lean to the side as you reach the opposite arm over. Hold for 10 seconds. Slowly straighten up, and repeat to the other side.

CONTINUED ▶

COOL-DOWN STRETCHES

Chest Stretch
Take your arms behind you and place one hand on top of the other. Raise your arms and feel the stretch across your chest. Hold for 10 seconds.

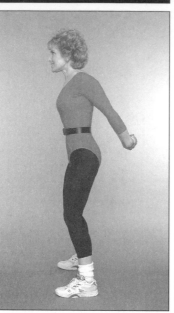

Front Thigh Stretch Hold on to the back of a chair. Keeping your inside leg slightly bent, bend the other leg and take hold of your foot. Ease the foot back and up, keeping both knees aligned. Hold for 10 seconds. Release, then turn round and repeat with the other leg.

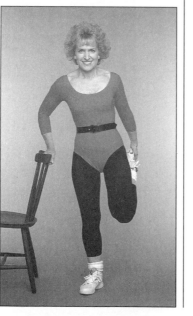

REVITALISER

With feet wide apart, bend your knees and make sweeping circles with your arms. Do 24.

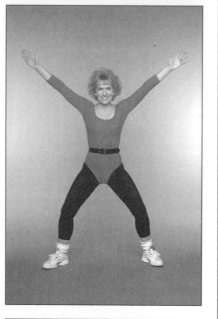

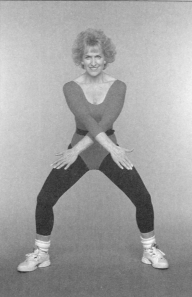

POSITIVE THOUGHT FOR THE DAY

I hope you are feeling good and in control. Your confidence should be growing by the day. Extra confidence should always be encouraged. It helps everyone around you.

Building a positive mental attitude within the family unit can be extremely beneficial for all concerned. If you don't already do it, make an effort to compliment children on a job well done, encourage them for trying hard at a particular task or project, and show an interest in what they do either at work or play. So often in personal relationships we get complacent about encouraging and complimenting our partners. We all have feelings and we all need positive encouragement. We should never take each other for granted. Ask yourself what you can do to make your partner's life more pleasant, more comfortable and less stressful. Working *with* your partner rather than against can produce such positive results that the whole relationship can grow remarkably, but trying to score points against them is futile.

It takes a confident person to compliment another but it really does promote a happier relationship. This in turn affects the whole family. Children who are conditioned in a positive environment will lead infinitely happier lives in later years.

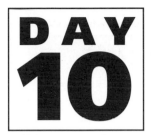

DAY 10

Day 10 and another day of achievement awaits you.

How are you progressing with your posture? Is pulling your tummy in and your shoulders back becoming more of a habit, and are you doing it for most of the day? Today, give it special attention and really make the effort to practise as often as possible.

Select menus that you enjoy and perform the exercises with particular care. If necessary re-read any instructions to ensure that you are executing them properly. Positioning yourself correctly can make all the difference to the effectiveness of any exercise. Really get into the momentum of the music as you practise.

When we follow a low-fat diet, going shopping can become quite an adventure. New products are constantly being introduced to the market, but beware! Clever marketing ploys entice us to buy products when the message on the label is not as clear as it might be. A product labelled 'low fat' might still be very high in fat. Low-fat spreads are a classic example. A full-fat butter or margarine is approximately 80 per cent fat. A low-fat brand could still be 40 per cent fat, which of course is still incredibly high. Look for products that contain four grams of fat or less per 100 grams of the total weight. It is easy to make mistakes, so check your labelling carefully. It doesn't matter what sort of fat it is – saturated or polyunsaturated. When we are talking about gaining body fat, all fat is the same. Look for the total number of fat grams and also work out the quantity of food you will be eating of that particular product. Four grams of fat per 100 grams equals 4 per cent fat. This is a good benchmark to use as a maximum. However, just because something has no fat in it does not necessarily mean that it is 'slimming'. Some sweets contain no fat, but they will cause you to gain weight because of their high calorie content. If you eat too much of anything, whether it be carbohydrate, protein or whatever, your body will convert what it doesn't need into fat. The only items you can consume freely that don't contain calories are items like water. Calories *do* count and we need to cut down our intake sufficiently to enable us to lose weight yet eat just enough to feed the body essential nutrients and allow it to work efficiently. If we eat too little, the body thinks it's going to be starved and its metabolism slows down. If we eat too much, we gain weight in the form of fat. Follow the diet as described and you'll get the balance just right. Have a great day today and be as physically active as you possibly can.

MENU

BREAKFAST

3 fl oz (75 ml) orange juice; 4 oz (100 g) low-fat cottage cheese mixed with 2 tsp strawberry jam; 1 piece fresh fruit
or
2 pieces fresh fruit; 2 x 5 oz (125 g) diet yogurts; 1 brown Ryvita spread with Marmite

LUNCH

P As much fresh fruit as you can eat at one sitting
1 x 5 oz (125 g) diet yogurt

Q ½ x 12 oz (300 g) can Campbell's Condensed Beef and Mushroom Soup reconstituted as directed; 2 slices light wholemeal bread, toasted (no butter); 1 piece fresh fruit

R *Chicken Tikka Pitta*
Split open 1 wholemeal pitta bread. Spread the inside with low-fat natural yogurt mixed with a little mint sauce. Fill with 3 oz (75 g) chicken tikka (ready prepared or homemade) and shredded salad

DINNER

STARTER
Triple Melon Salad
Fill a large to medium-sized individual glass dish with cubes of ogen, honeydew and water melons (10 oz/250 g total weight) and garnish with a sprig of mint

R 4 oz (100 g) roast lamb or beef served with the following: Dry-roast Potatoes (page 175); Dry-roast Parsnips (page 175); unlimited extra vegetables; gravy; mint sauce for the lamb and horseradish sauce for the beef

Q *Chicken Korma* (page 163)

V Batchelor's Beanfeast Soya Mince with Onion in a Savoury Gravy, served with unlimited potatoes and vegetables

DESSERT
Banana and Sultana Cake (page 178)

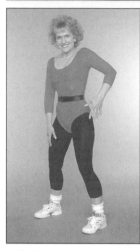

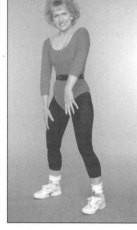

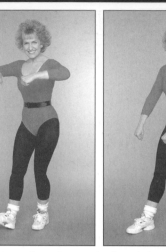

Roll alternate shoulders backwards, transferring your weight from one foot to the other. Do 16, then repeat, rolling shoulders forwards.

Tap the toes of one foot to the floor 8 times while punching down with your arms. Repeat with the other foot.

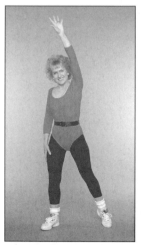

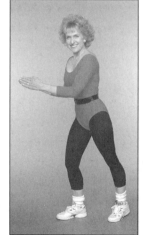

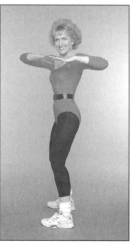

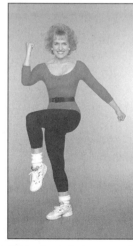

Transferring your weight from one foot to the other, swing alternate arms in complete circles. Do 16.

Take two steps to the side, moving your arms in a 'train-like' motion as you step. Repeat to the other side. Do 16 to alternate sides.

Keeping the hips square, twist your upper body from side to side. Do not jerk. Do 8 to each side.

Raise alternate knees and aim to touch with opposite elbow. Do 16.

Back of Thigh Stretch Bend one knee and, keeping your weight on that foot, extend the other leg in front, toes raised. Feel the stretch at the back of the knee and the thigh. Hold for 10 seconds, then change legs and repeat.

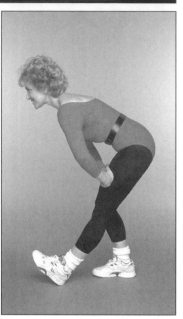

Calf Stretch Shift your weight on to the front leg and bend the knee. Your back leg is straight, heel on the floor and toes of both feet facing straight ahead. Keep your weight slightly forwards and feel the stretch in the calf muscle of your back leg. Hold for 10 seconds, then change legs and repeat.

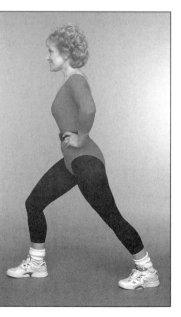

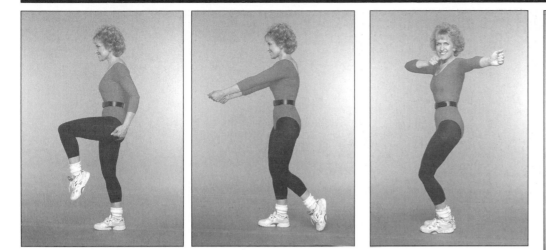

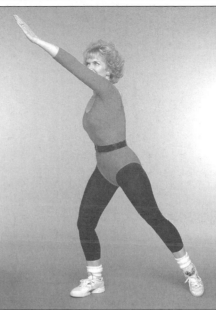

Step and lunge to one side, reaching across with opposite arm. Only the toes of the straight leg should touch the floor. Try to straighten the arm and leg as much as possible as you lunge. Repeat to the other side. Do 24 to alternate sides.

Raise one knee in front, then tap the toes behind, bringing the arms backwards and forwards as if pulling drawers out and in. Keep your tummy tight throughout. Do 24, then repeat with the other leg.

Bend your knees and pull an imaginary bow and arrow with your arms, then straighten the knees, and repeat to the other side. Do 24 to alternate sides.

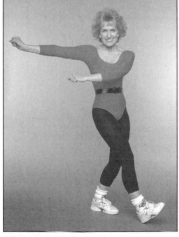

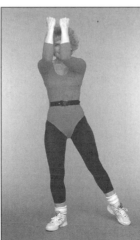

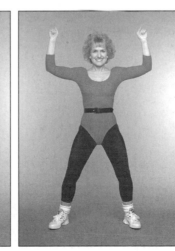

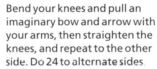

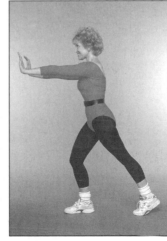

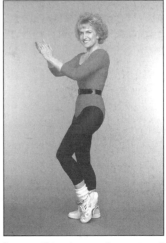

Swing alternate legs across and tap the floor with your heels, swinging your arms from side to side as you step. Do 16.

With feet wide apart, step and touch alternate feet to the side, bringing your bent elbows in and out at shoulder level. Do 24.

Step and touch the floor behind with alternate feet, pushing your hands forwards as you take each foot back. Do 32.

Do a walking jog on the spot and clap your hands in front. Do 16.

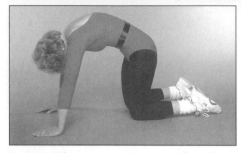

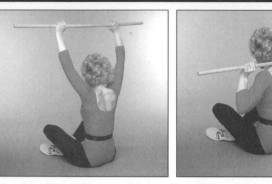

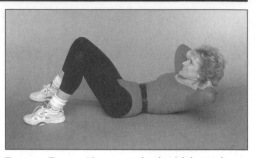

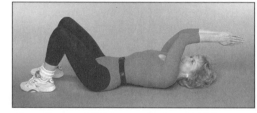

Tummy Trimmer Position yourself on all fours and pull your tummy muscles in as tightly as you can to arch your spine. Relax, and repeat 14–16 times.

Shoulder Strengthener Take a pole and sit upright in a comfortable position. Raise the pole above your head, then lower it, squeezing your shoulder blades together. Repeat. Do 14–16, concentrating on bringing your shoulder blades together as you lower the pole.

Tummy Toner Lie on your back with knees bent and your *tummy pulled in tightly*. Place your hands behind your neck and slowly raise your head and shoulders off the floor. Raise on a count of 2, then return to the floor on a count of 2. Do 14–16.

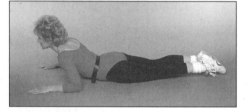

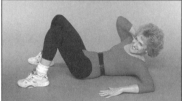

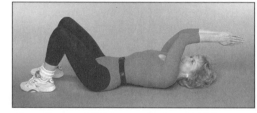

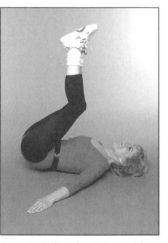

Back Strengthener Lie face down with arms bent, palms facing upwards. Slowly raise your chest off the floor, using the muscles in your back not your arms. Return to the floor and repeat. Do 14–16.

Waist Toner Lie on your back with knees bent. Place one hand behind your neck and have the other arm on the floor for support. Raise the head and shoulder and bring your elbow towards the opposite knee, taking care not to roll your hips. Return to the floor, and repeat. Do 14–16, then repeat to the other side.

Chest Toner Still lying on the floor with knees bent, place your arms out to the sides with elbows bent at shoulder level. Lift your arms and press the elbows and palms together. Keeping the arms together and parallel with the floor, push them over your head and then pull them forwards again. Repeat this backwards and forwards movement 14–16 times, keeping the elbows together throughout the exercise.

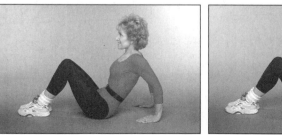

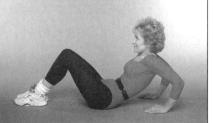

Upper Arm Toner Sit with knees bent and prop yourself up on your hands. Your hands should be placed at least 12 inches (30 cm) behind your back, with fingers pointing forwards. Bend your arms so that your elbows move backwards, then straighten them again. Do 12–14.

Tummy Trimmer Lying with legs raised and slightly bent, press your tummy muscles down and lift the hips slightly off the floor. Repeat 10–12 times, ensuring the effort comes from your abdomen, not your arms.

COOL-DOWN STRETCHES

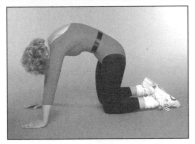

Back Stretch Position yourself on all fours and arch the spine as much as possible, pulling the tummy towards the spine. Hold for 10 seconds.

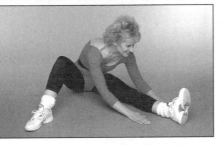

Back of the Thigh Stretch Sitting with one leg straight and the other slightly bent, ease your weight forwards towards the straight leg and feel the stretch at the back of the knee and thigh. Hold for 10 seconds, then change position and repeat with the other leg.

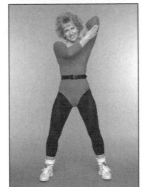

Back of Upper Arm Stretch Stand with feet a comfortable distance apart and knees slightly bent. Raise one elbow and ease your hand down your back, using the other arm to assist. Hold for 10 seconds. Relax, and repeat with the other arm.

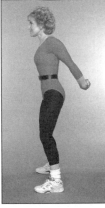

Chest Stretch Stand with feet a comfortable distance apart and knees slightly bent. Take your arms behind you and place one hand on top of the other. Raise your arms to expand your chest. Feel the stretch across your chest. Hold for 10 seconds.

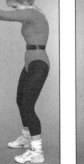

Upper Back Stretch Round your back and raise your arms in front to shoulder level to separate your shoulder blades. Hold for 10 seconds.

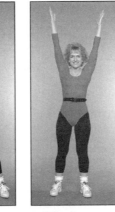

Waist Stretch Place one hand on your thigh for support and lean to the side as you reach the opposite arm over. Hold for 10 seconds. Slowly straighten up, and repeat to the other side.

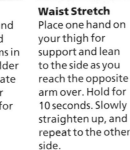

Full Body Stretch Standing upright, reach your arms towards the ceiling and hold for 10 seconds.

REVITALISER

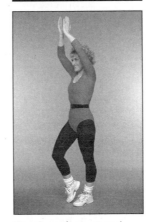

March on the spot and clap your hands above your head. Do 32.

POSITIVE THOUGHT FOR THE DAY

Developing a positive mental attitude can take on many aspects. Making people feel important reaps wonderful rewards and enables us to get the very best out of those with whom we live and work. Being interested in other people and being able to listen to their fears as well as their dreams can make all the difference to how they feel about their lives. But we all need to have a goal. That goal may be losing weight and getting into better physical shape, but we should also think about long-term, tangible goals. Things that we can work towards and give us a reason for trying our very best at what we do. If we don't have a good reason for doing something, then it is unlikely that we will give our best performance. Yes, of course, pride does matter, but pride alone may not be enough. It's good to understand what we all mean by success, but we must decide what success means for us personally and not what someone else deems it to be. Every one of us has the equipment to achieve whatever it is we really want to achieve. But, sadly, so few people have any real idea of what they want out of life. I ask you now to seriously think about what you would like out of life – in three weeks' time, in three months' time and in three years' time. Think about it and write it down in a diary. Keep going back to it and amending it, as your goals may change. If you aim for something that is really quite ambitious, undoubtedly, you would achieve a higher goal than if you went for something that is well within your reach, even if you don't actually reach your ultimate goal. Remember, for a goal to be worth working for, it must be great enough to warrant the extra effort. It must also be realistic. Plan your first goal today and make sure it can be achieved within three months. As we achieve goals our confidence grows and we are able to achieve more and more.

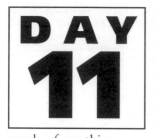

DAY 11

I hope you got on well yesterday and were able to do all the exercises and stick rigidly to the diet. Yesterday we looked at how calories do count and how, if we consume too much of anything, we convert any excess into fat. I am often asked if it is possible to save up the daily alcohol allowance and have a real binge at the weekend. If you want to lose weight, then I'm afraid you can't. Alcohol contains a significant amount of sugar. Whilst I am not against having a tiny amount of sugar in our daily diet, to have it in excess is only going to lead to it being laid down as fat. One alcoholic drink a day will soon be utilised by the body, and the calories that it provides will be burned away within an hour or two. On the other hand, if we consume excessive amounts, any calories not used by the body will be converted straight into fat. This means that one drinking binge could effectively undo a great deal of the good that you have achieved on this programme. Men are allowed two drinks per day because of their size, but men who drink a lot of alcohol often end up with large stomachs where the fat has been created by the excess alcohol. To have an occasional drink on a diet is, I believe, both enjoyable and helpful. It is sociable and helps us forget that we are on a diet. The fewer drastic changes we have to make in the way we eat and live our everyday lives, the greater our chances of long-term success.

Select your various meals with care today and put as much effort as you can into your exercise session. Remember to be as physically active as you can and realise the benefits that you are achieving in doing so. Enjoy your drink tonight. Cheers!

MENU

BREAKFAST

1¹/₂ oz (37.5 g) muesli topped with 4 oz (100 g) fresh fruit, e.g. strawberries, mixed with 5 oz (125 g) diet yogurt, any flavour

or

¹/₄ pint/5 fl oz (125 ml) orange or grapefruit juice 2 slices wholemeal toast spread with 3 tsp marmalade; 1 x 5 oz (125 g) diet yogurt

LUNCH

P **Curried Prawn Cocktail Sandwich**
Mix together 1 tbsp low-calorie salad dressing and ¹/₂ tsp curry paste and spread on to 2 slices wholemeal bread. Fill with shredded lettuce and 3 oz (75 g) prawns

Q 8 oz (200 g) jacket potato topped with 3 oz (75 g) low-fat coleslaw, plus 10 sultanas and salad; 1 x 5 oz (125 g) diet yogurt

R **Carrot and Tarragon Soup** (page 157)
plus 1 slice wholemeal bread (no butter)

DINNER

STARTER
4 oz (100 g) melon and 4 oz (100 g) strawberries

R **Tandoori Chicken Thatch** (page 165)

Q Findus Lean Cuisine Chicken and Ham Lasagne Verdi, served with additional vegetables

V **Cabbage and Leek Bake** (page 170)

DESSERT
2 brown Ryvitas spread with Marmite and 3 oz (75 g) low-fat cottage cheese

WARM-UP

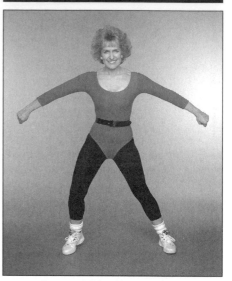

Take two steps to the side, swinging arms in and out as you step. Repeat to the other side. Do 24 to alternate sides.

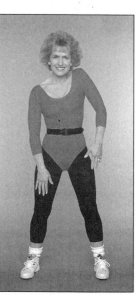

With feet hip-width apart and knees slightly bent, shrug alternate shoulders 16 times.

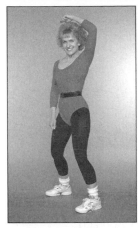

Rotate alternate arms back-wards as if brushing your hair, transferring your weight from one foot to the other. Do 16.

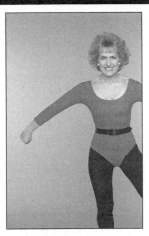

Extend alternate legs to the side, tapping the toes to the floor as you step. Do 16.

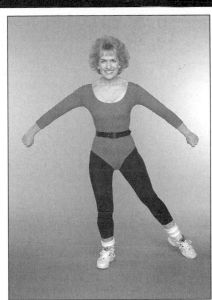

Extend alternate legs to the side, pointing your toes and swinging your arms in and out as you step. Do 16.

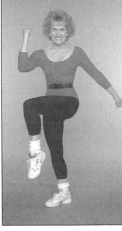

Raise alternate knees across and aim to touch with opposite elbow. Keep your tummy pulled in and your back straight. Do 24.

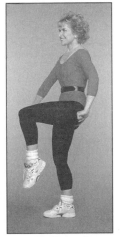

Raise alternate knees in front, pressing down with both arms. Keep your tummy tight and back straight. Do 16.

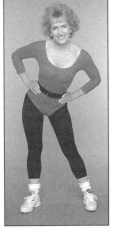

Rotate your hips in a clockwise direction. Do 8, then repeat in an anti-clockwise direction.

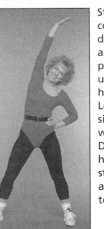

Stand with feet a comfortable distance apart, one arm raised with palm facing upwards, the other hand on your hip. Lean directly to the side, reaching over with the raised arm. Do not twist the hips. Return to the starting position, and repeat. Do 16 to alternate sides.

Back of Thigh Stretch
Bend one knee and, keeping your weight on that foot, extend the other leg in front, toes raised. Feel the stretch at the back of the knee and the thigh. Hold for 10 seconds, then change legs and repeat.

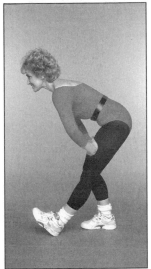

Calf Stretch
Shift your weight on to the front leg and bend the knee. Your back leg is straight, heel on the floor and toes of both feet facing straight ahead. Keep your weight slightly forwards and feel the stretch in the calf muscle of your back leg. Hold for 10 seconds, then change legs and repeat.

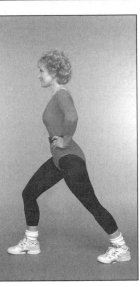

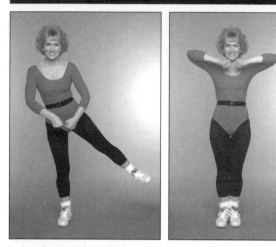 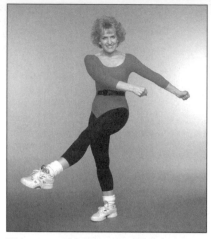 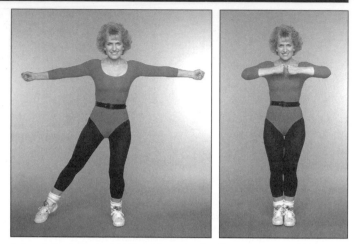

Raise alternate legs to the side, keeping your hips square and bending and straightening both arms in front. Do 32.

Kick across with alternate feet, swinging your arms from side to side. Do 32.

Extend alternate feet to the side, swinging the arms out and in at shoulder level. Do 32.

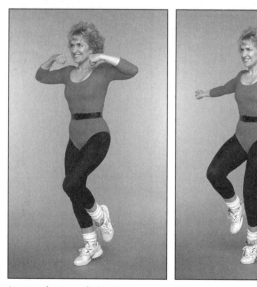 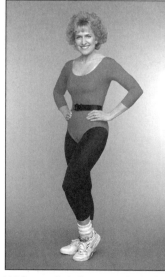 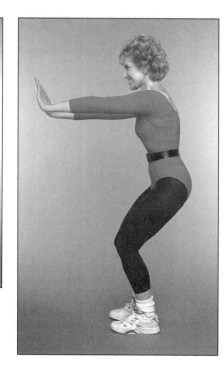

Bend your knees, pushing your arms forwards. Straighten them again and bring your arms backwards. Do 32.

Jog on the spot, bringing your arms in and out at shoulder level. Do 32.

With your hands on your hips, do a walking jog on the spot. Do 32.

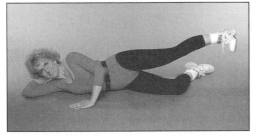

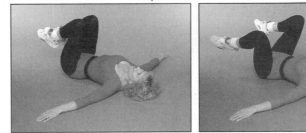

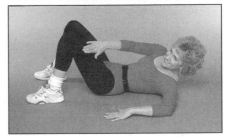

Outer Thigh Toner Lie on your side with your bottom leg bent and your top leg straight. Raise the top leg, keeping your hips square and your toes aiming slightly downwards. Do not raise the leg too high. Lower, then repeat. Do 12–14, then roll over and repeat with the other leg.

Inner Thigh Toner Lying on your back with your knees bent and raised over your hips, separate your knees and then bring them together again, keeping your back pressed into the floor. Do 12–14.

Waist Toner Supporting yourself with one arm, reach across your body with the other arm, pressing your tummy down as you reach. Take care not to roll the hips. Return to the floor, and repeat. Do 12–14, then repeat to the other side.

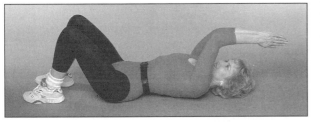

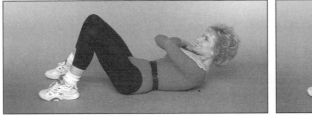

Chest Toner Lie on your back with knees bent and place your arms out to the sides with elbows bent at shoulder level. Lift your arms and press the elbows and palms together. Keeping the arms together and parallel with the floor, push them over your head and then pull them forwards again. Repeat this backwards and forwards movement 12–14 times, keeping the elbows together throughout the exercise.

Tummy Toner Lie on your back with your knees bent and your hands placed across your chest. Support your neck with one hand if you prefer. *Pulling your tummy in tightly*, raise your head and shoulders off the floor for a count of 2, then lower to a count of 2. Keep a distance between your chin and your chest. Breathe out as you come up and breathe in as you go down. Do 12–14.

Outer Thigh Toner Lie on your side with both knees slightly bent. Dip the knee of the top leg on the floor in front and then, leading with the heel, extend and straighten it towards the corner of the room. Repeat this dipping and straightening movement 8 times, ensuring the hips remain square. Roll over, and repeat with the other leg.

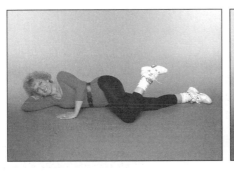

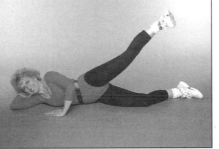

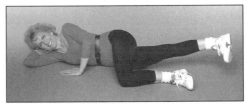

Inner Thigh Toner Bend the top leg and rest it on the floor, in front of you. Keeping the bottom leg straight, lift it up and down 12–14 times. Roll over, and repeat with the other leg.

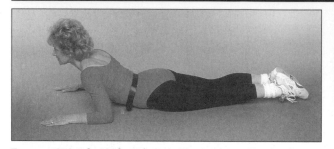

Tummy Stretch Lie face down with arms bent. Slowly raise your head and shoulders off the floor, supporting yourself on your forearms and elbows, and feel the stretch down the front of your abdomen. Hold for 10 seconds.

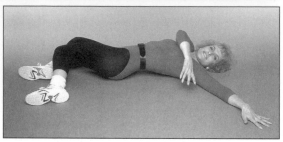

Waist and Outer Thigh Stretch Lie on your back with both knees bent. Allow your knees to drop to one side while taking your arms to the opposite side. Hold for 10 seconds, then slowly return to the centre, and repeat to the other side.

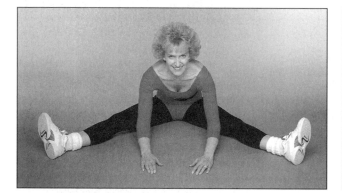

Advanced Inner Thigh Stretch Sitting with your legs wide apart and supporting your weight on your arms, ease your body forwards and feel the stretch in your inner thighs. Hold for 10 seconds.

Chest Stretch Sitting with legs crossed, raise your arms and clasp your hands behind your back to stretch the muscles across your chest. Hold for 10 seconds.

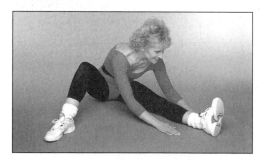

Back of Thigh Stretch Sitting with one leg straight and the other slightly bent, ease your weight forwards towards the straight leg and feel the stretch at the back of the knee and the thigh. Hold for 10 seconds, then change the position of the legs to repeat on the other side.

POSITIVE THOUGHT FOR THE DAY

I hope you had a chance to plan your goals for the next few months. Perhaps you managed to determine a long-term goal for which you can work over the next few years. It is really helpful if you can discuss your goals with your partner. If two people agree on their goals and are pulling in the same direction then you just can't fail. My husband Mike and I work together on our goals and it works brilliantly. We wouldn't be where we are today if we didn't.

You now need to define your goals a little more clearly. Make a list of all the various aspects of achieving each goal and the timetable that will be required to achieve it. It's all about having a purpose and having something to look forward to. People don't plan to fail but they do fail to plan and unless we have something *to* plan and work towards we will not achieve anything. We need to ask ourselves if we are going to guide our lives towards the goals that we want or just allow them to drift any old way and achieve nothing. When setting your goal, start off with the most basic needs and work up from there. Once you have completed your list you can sit back and relax. Just start with the first item on the list and when you have done it, tick it off and then go on to the next. You don't have to worry yet about items further down the list. Just think of the next stage. However, each stage needs to be clearly defined, so bear this in mind in your planning.

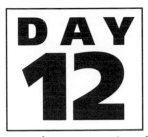

DAY 12

Well done for getting this far. You are now nearing the end of this second week and you should be feeling significantly slimmer and fitter. Try on your skirt or pair of trousers again today and see how much looser it is. If you are finding the going is getting a bit tough, remember, anything worth working for doesn't come instantly. Never is this more true than with regard to trimness and fitness. Just as we didn't become overweight and unfit overnight, nor should we expect to remedy the situation overnight either. The good news is that we will be able to make faster progress in getting the excess weight off and increasing our fitness than the time it took to get us into that sorry state in the first place. Furthermore, it doesn't matter what age we are when we start. In terms of fitness an 80-year-old will make progress just as fast as a 20-year-old, and recent trials have proved that when older people become more physically active, their mental alertness improves too.

If you can motivate yourself to lead a more active life, you will find that the more you do the more you will be able to do. People who are physically fit are far less likely to suffer from depression, they recover from illnesses more quickly and are less likely to be stressed. Fit people get much more out of life. You have made a very important step towards improving your life. Keep going. Continue to enjoy the benefits and watch yourself getting younger as you get older! Be good today. You only have two more days before weighing and measuring day. Stick on in there!

MENU

BREAKFAST

6 oz (150 g) any canned fruit in natural juice topped with 5 oz (125 g) diet yogurt

or

¼ pint/5 fl oz (125 ml) orange juice; 2 oz (50 g) smoked turkey breast, fresh sliced tomatoes, plus 1 wholemeal roll (2 oz/50 g) spread with horseradish sauce

LUNCH

P 4 slices light bread spread with a little jam and filled with 1 mashed banana; 1 x 8 oz (200 g) pot Müllerlight yogurt

Q 4 brown Ryvitas spread with 2½ oz (62.5 g) Princes Mackerel Fillets in Spicy Tomato Sauce mixed with 2 tsp horseradish sauce plus 2 pieces fresh fruit

R *Chicken and Sweetcorn Soup* (page 158) plus 1 slice wholemeal bread (no butter)

DINNER

STARTER
Garlic and Mint Yogurt Dip with Crudités (page157)

R *Chicken Madras* (page 164)

Q *Spicy Sweet and Sour Chicken or Pork with Crispy Vegetables* (page 166)

V *Vegetable Curry* (page 173)

DESSERT
Fresh Fruit Salad (page 176)

WARM-UP

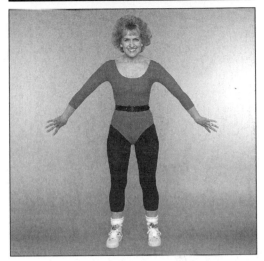

With arms out to the sides, rotate your arms forwards and backwards. Do 8

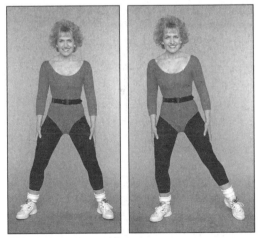

With feet a comfortable distance apart, transfer your weight from one foot to the other, bending your knees and tapping the toes of the opposite foot as you step. Do 16.

CONTINUED ▶

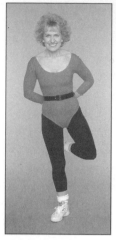
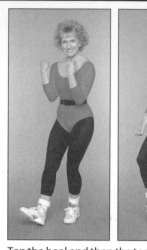
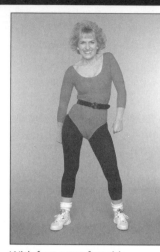
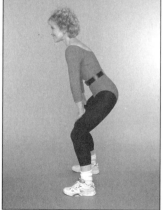
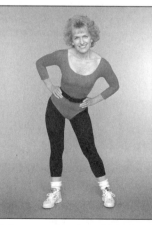

Kick back with alternate feet. Do 16.

Tap the heel and then the toe of one foot, flexing and straightening both arms. Do 8, then repeat with the other foot. Repeat again with each foot.

With feet a comfortable distance apart, raise one hip and at the same time raise the opposite shoulder. Repeat with the other hip and shoulder. Do 16 on alternate sides.

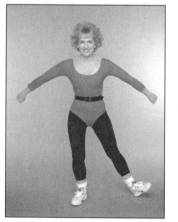

Extend alternate legs to the side, tapping the floor with your heels and swinging your arms in and out. Do 16.

With feet wide apart, bend your knees and go down into a squat, making sure the knees bend over the ankles. Come up again, and repeat. Do 8.

Rotate your hips in a clockwise direction. Do 8, then repeat in an anti-clockwise direction.

Back of Thigh Stretch Bend one knee and, keeping your weight on that foot, extend the other leg in front, toes raised. Feel the stretch at the back of the knee and the thigh. Hold for 10 seconds, then change legs and repeat.

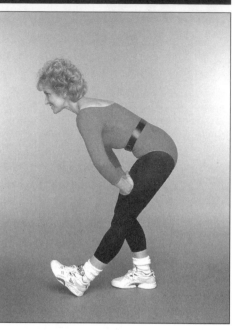

Calf Stretch Shift your weight on to the front leg and bend the knee. Your back leg is straight, heel on the floor and toes of both feet facing straight ahead. Keep your weight slightly forwards and feel the stretch in the calf muscle of your back leg. Hold for 10 seconds, then change legs and repeat.

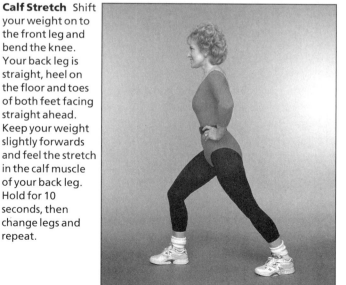

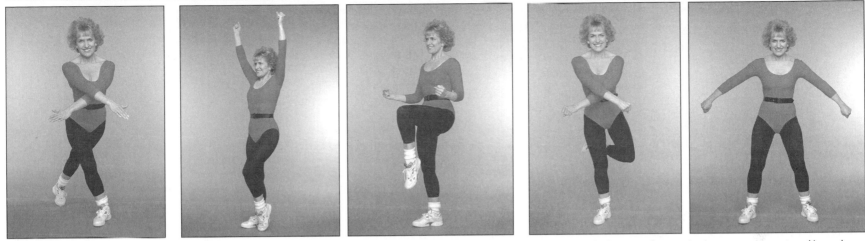

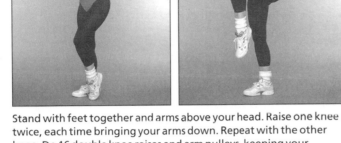

Step to the side and curtsey with one leg behind, swinging your arms out to the side and crossing them in front as you step. Do 32.

Stand with feet together and arms above your head. Raise one knee twice, each time bringing your arms down. Repeat with the other knee. Do 16 double knee raises and arm pulleys, keeping your tummy tight throughout.

Kick back with alternate feet, swinging your arms out and in and crossing them in front. Do 32.

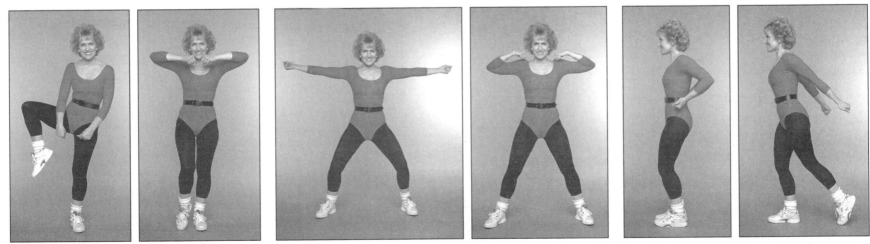

Raise alternate knees out to the side, pushing your arms down and up in 'barrow boy' style as you step. Do 32.

With feet wide apart, toes and knees facing slightly outwards, squat down, then come up again, bending and straightening your arms at shoulder level as you squat. Do 8.

Tap alternate feet behind you, extending your arms to the back. Keep your elbows as far back and as close together as possible throughout. Do 32.

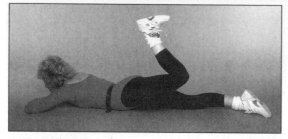

Back of Thigh Toner Lie on your front and rest your head on your hands. Bend one leg and push the heel towards the ceiling, extending the leg slightly as you do so. Do 12–14, then repeat with the other leg.

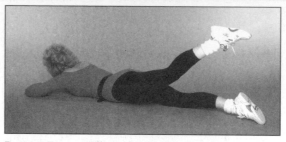

Bottom Toner Still resting your head on your hands, raise one leg straight up and down, squeezing your seat as you raise. Keep your hips pressed into the floor throughout. Do 12–14, then repeat with the other leg.

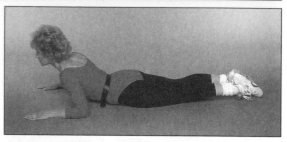

Back Strengthener Place your arms to the sides with elbows bent, palms facing upwards. Slowly raise your chest off the floor, using the muscles in your back not your arms. Return to the floor and repeat. Do 12–14.

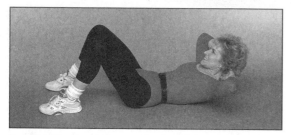

Tummy Toner Lie on your back with knees bent and your *tummy pulled in tightly*. Place your hands behind your neck and slowly raise your head and shoulders off the floor. Raise on a count of 2, then return to the floor on a count of 2. Do 14–16.

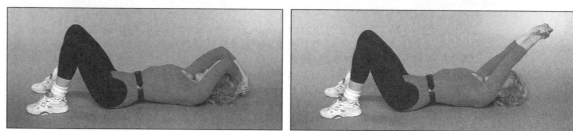

Upper Arm Toner Bend your arms and place them over your head. Straighten the arms, then bend them again. Repeat this movement 16–18 times.

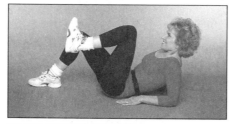

Front Thigh Toner Supporting yourself on your arms, bend both knees. Bring one knee in towards your chest and then extend the leg straight out in front. Keep your tummy tight to support your back. Bring the leg towards your chest again, and repeat. Do 12–14, then repeat with the other leg.

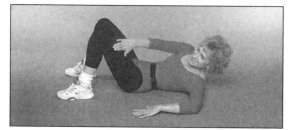

Waist Toner Lie back on the floor. Supporting yourself with one arm, reach across your body with the other arm, pressing your tummy down as you reach. Take care not to roll the hips. Return to the floor, and repeat. Do 14–16, then repeat to the other side.

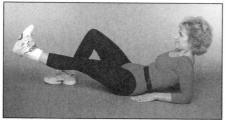

Tummy Trimmer Lie on your back with legs raised and slightly bent. Your feet are over your hips and your tummy is pulled in tightly. Press your tummy muscles down and lift the hips slightly off the floor. Repeat 10–12 times, ensuring the effort comes from your abdomen, not your arms.

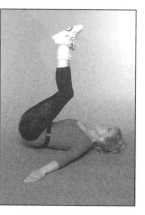

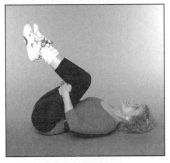

Seat Stretch Still lying on your back with knees towards your chest, place your hands underneath your thighs. Ease your legs further towards your chest and feel the stretch in your seat. Hold for 10 seconds.

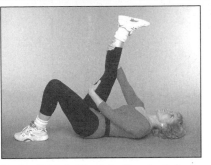

Back of Thigh Stretch Place both feet on the floor. Take hold of one leg and raise it, straightening it as far as is comfortable. Ease the leg towards you with your hands and hold for 10–15 seconds. Relax, and repeat with the other leg.

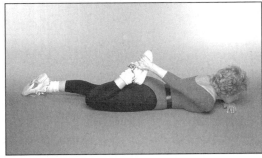

Front Thigh Stretch Lie face down and rest your face on one hand. Bend the opposite leg and use your hand to ease it towards your seat. Hold for 10 seconds then release, and repeat with the other leg.

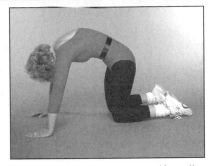

Back Stretch Position yourself on all fours and arch the spine as much as possible, pulling your tummy towards your spine. Hold for 10 seconds.

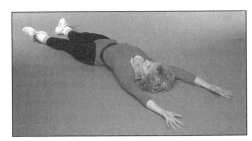

Full Body Stretch Lie on your back and extend your arms and legs as much as possible. Hold for 10 seconds.

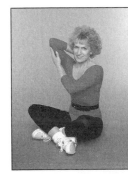

Back of Upper Arm Stretch Sit up with legs crossed. Raise one elbow and ease your hand down your back. Use the other arm to ease it further. Hold for 10 seconds. Repeat with the other arm.

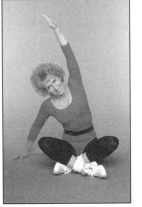

Waist Stretch Place one hand on the floor for support, and reach over to the side with the other arm. Hold for 10 seconds, then relax and repeat to the other side.

POSITIVE THOUGHT FOR THE DAY

Many of the ideas on adopting a positive attitude and achieving goals that I have included in this book are ones I have learned from a variety of books and motivational tapes. All have been tested and proved to be effective. I use them all the time, and I hope you are finding them helpful too.

Another idea for building confidence is to compile a record of past successes and goals achieved. Keep a notebook and write down, for instance, a nice comment that somebody made to you, or include a letter you have received in which someone has written kind words about you. It is always good to be able to refer back to our 'confidence book' on those days when we feel lacking in confidence and not very happy about ourselves. We all have those kinds of days – they are part of life. But being able to remember the nice things that people have said to us can be such a comfort. Unfortunately, all too often we remember only the cutting remarks and the criticisms, rather than the compliments. If we keep a written record of these compliments, we can recharge our confidence battery by referring back to them. So today, find yourself a notebook or scrapbook and, from now on, start noting down comments that people make about how much slimmer and healthier you look. Write down your own comments too about how much more confident you feel, how much more energy you have and how successful you have been on this diet and exercise programme. It is worth the effort and will help you through the sticky times. Just remember, no one else need ever read it. This is just for you.

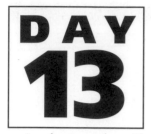

DAY 13

You are nearly at the end of your second week and you need to pump up your willpower supply so that you don't cheat when weighing and measuring day is so close. Try on the 'measuring' skirt or trousers and see and feel the difference. The inches should really be disappearing by now. Fill yourself up with lots of low-calorie diet drinks, and don't eat *anything* between meals. Stick to the menus for today and fill up on vegetables if you feel peckish at meal times. The rewards are so great that moments of strong willpower now will prove *so* worthwhile when you get on the scales the day after tomorrow. Don't even *think* about cheating! If you are going to succeed you need to make sacrifices, but, believe me, they are worth working for.

How are you getting on with the exercises? Remember to adjust the number of repetitions in the aerobic and toning exercises to suit your ability. If you are finding them too easy you should increase the repetitions in order to challenge your body further and obtain greater benefits. But remember, the aim is to reach the point of fatigue, not pain.

Have a terrific day and feel very virtuous this evening.

MENU

BREAKFAST

5 prunes soaked in tea overnight and served with
2 tsp low-fat fromage frais or yogurt

or

4 fl oz (100 ml) orange juice; 1 slice (1½ oz/37.5 g)
wholemeal toast topped with 1 x 8 oz (200 g) can tomatoes,
well seasoned and cooked until juice has thickened
1 x 5 oz (125 g) diet yogurt

LUNCH

P Salmon and Watercress Sandwich

Spread 2 slices wholemeal bread with reduced-oil salad
dressing. Mix ½ bunch chopped watercress leaves with
2 tbsp reduced-oil salad dressing and a little lemon juice.
Mix with 2 oz (50 g) chunks of lightly cooked fresh or canned
salmon. Spread on to the bread, garnish with watercress and
cucumber and serve as an open or closed sandwich

Q Chicken Leg with Salad

6 oz (150 g) chicken leg (weighed with bone) with
all skin removed, served with mixed salad,
2 oz (50 g) Branston pickle and oil-free salad dressing
1 x 8 oz (200 g) pot Müllerlight yogurt

R Tuna and Sweetcorn Cakes (page 169)

DINNER

STARTER
Cheesy Pears (page 156)

R Chicken and Mushroom Bake (page 164)

Q 4 oz (100 g) lean steak, grilled and served with
8 oz (200 g) jacket potato or new potatoes topped with
3 oz (75 g) low-fat fromage frais and unlimited vegetables

V Stuffed Marrow (page 171)

DESSERT
Kiwi Fruit Mousse (page 177)

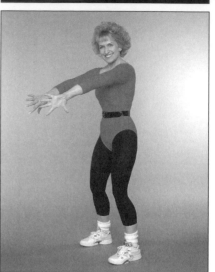

Standing with arms out in front, rotate arms inwards and outwards 8 times.

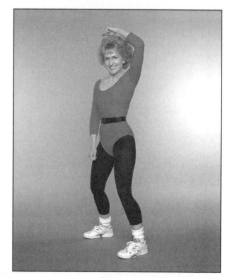

Rotate alternate arms backwards as if brushing your hair, transferring your weight from one foot to the other. Do 16.

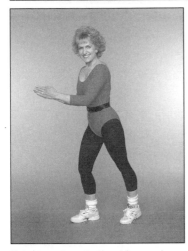

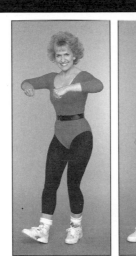

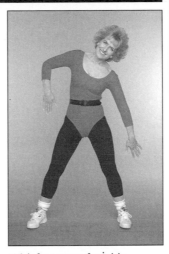

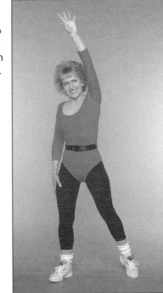

Take two steps to the side, moving your arms in a 'train-like' motion as you step. Repeat to the other side. Do 16 to alternate sides.

Tap the toes of one foot to the floor 8 times while punching down with your arms. Repeat with the other foot. Repeat again with each foot.

With feet a comfortable distance apart, lean over to the side without twisting the hips. Repeat to the other side. Do 8 to each side.

Back of Thigh Stretch Bend one knee and, keeping your weight on that foot, extend the other leg in front, toes raised. Feel the stretch at the back of the knee and the thigh. Hold for 10 seconds, then change legs and repeat.

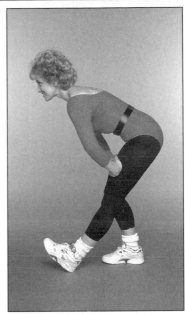

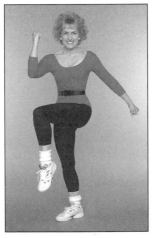

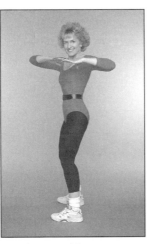

Transferring your weight from one foot to the other, swing alternate arms in complete circles. Do 16.

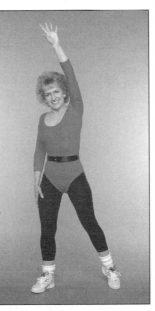

Calf Stretch Shift your weight on to the front leg and bend the knee. Your back leg is straight, heel on the floor and toes of both feet facing straight ahead. Keep your weight slightly forwards and feel the stretch in the calf muscle of your back leg. Hold for 10 seconds, then change legs and repeat.

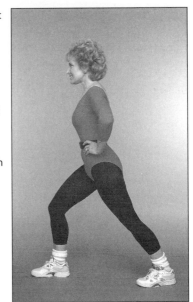

Raise alternate knees and aim to touch with opposite elbow. Keep the tummy tight. Do 32.

Keeping your hips square, twist your upper body from side to side. Do not jerk. Do 8 to each side.

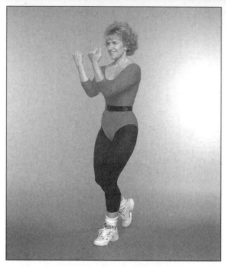

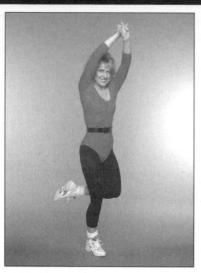

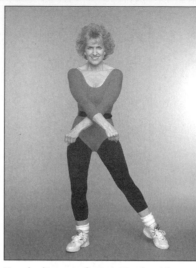

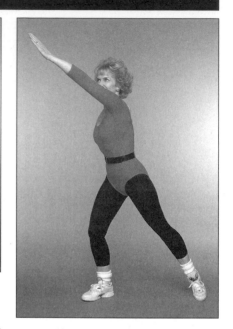

Step and touch the floor behind with alternate feet, flexing and straightening your arms as you step. Do 32.

Kick back with alternate feet, swinging your arms out and in to cross overhead. Do 32.

Touch alternate feet out to the side, swinging your arms out and in to cross in front. Do 32.

Step and lunge to one side, reaching across with opposite arm. Only the toes of the straight leg should touch the floor. Try to straighten the arm and leg as much as possible as you lunge. Repeat to the other side. Do 32 to alternate sides.

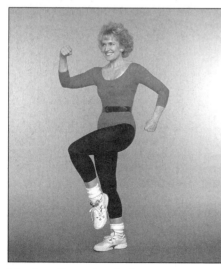

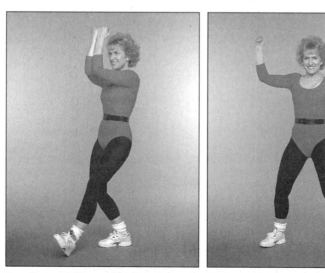

March on the spot, swinging your arms strongly. Don't stamp. Do 32.

Standing with feet wide apart, swing one leg across and tap your heel to the floor, taking your bent arms in and out at shoulder level as you step. Repeat with the other foot. Do 32 with alternate feet.

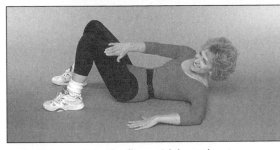

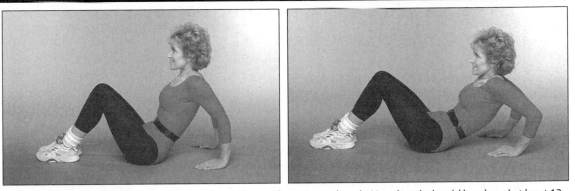

Waist Toner Lie on the floor with knees bent. Supporting yourself with one arm, reach across your body with the other arm, pressing your tummy down as you reach. Take care not to roll the hips. Return to the floor, and repeat. Do 14–16, then repeat to the other side.

Upper Arm Toner Sit with knees bent and prop yourself up on your hands. Your hands should be placed at least 12 inches (30 cm) behind your back, with fingers pointing forwards. Bend your arms so that your elbows move backwards, then straighten them again. Do 12–14.

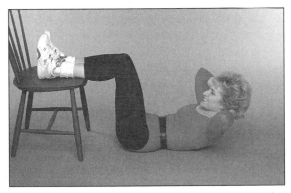

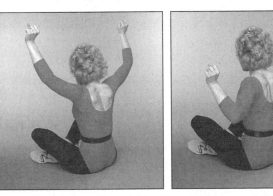

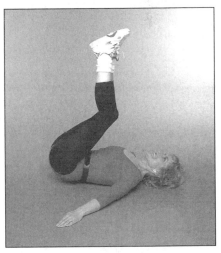

Tummy Toner Lie on your back with your feet placed against a wall or on a sturdy chair, and support your head with your hands. *Pulling your tummy in tightly*, raise your head and shoulders off the floor, keeping a distance between your chin and your chest. Raise on a count of 2, and return to the floor on a count of 2. Repeat 14–16 times.

Upper Back Toner Sit upright with your legs crossed. Take your arms above your head and reach up. Now pull the elbows back and down to squeeze your shoulder blades together. Raise the arms again, and repeat. Do 12–14.

Tummy Trimmer Lying with legs raised and slightly bent, press your tummy muscles down and lift the hips slightly off the floor. Repeat 12–14 times, ensuring the effort comes from your abdomen, not your arms.

Back Strengthener Lie face down with arms bent, palms facing upwards. Slowly raise your chest off the floor, using the muscles in your back not your arms. Return to the floor and repeat. Do 10–12.

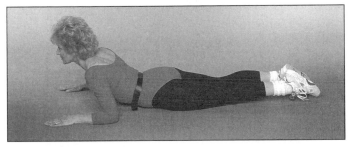

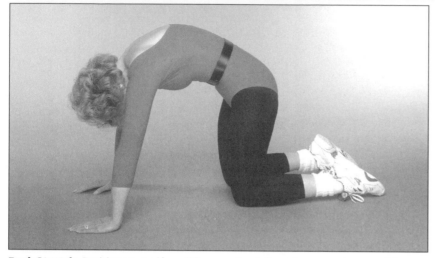

Back Stretch Position yourself on all fours and arch the spine as much as possible, pulling the tummy towards the spine. Hold for 10 seconds.

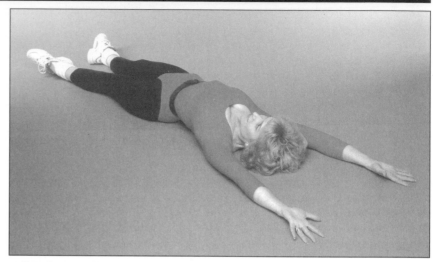

Full Body Stretch Lie on your back and extend your arms and legs as much as possible. Hold for 10 seconds.

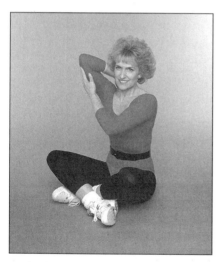

Back of Upper Arm Stretch Sit up with legs crossed. Raise one elbow and ease your hand down your back. Use the other arm to ease it further. Hold for 10 seconds. Repeat with the other arm.

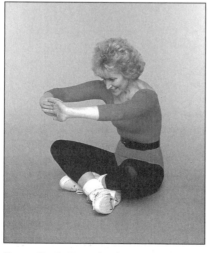

Upper Back Stretch Sitting with legs crossed, round your back and raise your arms in front to shoulder level to separate your shoulder blades. Hold for 10 seconds.

POSITIVE THOUGHT FOR THE DAY

I hope you have had a good day and are feeling strong and confident. Are those around you helping or hindering your progress?

In our daily lives, we inevitably mix with many people from different environments. Where they work, live or where they come from is irrelevant, but their attitude is very important. People who have a negative outlook are usually miserable, they worry a lot, they have no goals or plans, they fear failure and they always have problems in life and blame others when things go wrong. They often cheat themselves and they try to destroy other people's hopes and dreams. They can cause so much damage to our personalities and our lives. On the other hand, positive people are happy, enthusiastic, they do have goals and they do have plans. They are self-confident and they have an expanding minds. If something goes wrong they look at themselves, not others, and try to work out why they went wrong. They are honest about their own strengths and weaknesses and, instead of tearing down other people's hopes and dreams, they help them to build them. Are you a positive or a negative person? Are those with whom you mix positive or negative? Do you need to make some changes?

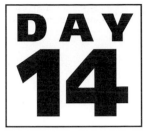

DAY 14

Congratulations, you've reached the end of Week 2. Make the most of today and try to be saintly with the diet and extra energetic with your activities. It's only 24 hours before you weigh and measure yourself for your second progress report. Let's make it a stunning success. Prepare yourself for the fact that you may not have lost as much weight during the second week but, hopefully, many inches will have disappeared – and that's what really matters. Work hard on your posture today, walk tall, concentrate on pulling in that tummy and enjoy the fact that your waist is significantly 'narrower' than it was two weeks ago. Cast your eye over the menus of the last seven days and place a tick alongside any particular recipes that you really enjoyed and would like to use again. Try them again next week and make the diet work for you. Encourage your family to be more physically active and involve them in sporting activities. Play ball with the younger children. Why not have a go at football, cricket, tennis or rounders? Swimming is a wonderfully positive activity as it not only helps you to burn fat and get fitter, it may even be a lifesaver. Over the last two weeks you have made real strides towards being healthier. Make activity a way of life from now on.

Your abdomen should be significantly flatter than it was two weeks ago. In two weeks' time it will be flatter still. It is particularly important for us to lose weight from around our abdominal area if that is where we carry our excess fat. The risk of cardiovascular disease is greater in those people who lay down excess body fat in that area. This is why men, generally, are at greater risk of stroke or heart disease, but women who tend to store fat in the abdominal area are at risk too. Although this diet and exercise plan has been specifically designed to help reduce fat in the abdominal area, when we follow a low-fat diet we lose fat from a variety of areas on our bodies. The good news is that, unlike most calorie-controlled diets that include fat, we lose it first from those fatty areas where we need to lose it most. By the end of today you will be halfway towards your goal of completing this 28-day programme. You will have reduced the fat on your body, increased your lean muscle mass, and you will be much fitter. Keep going forward and don't look back.

MENU

BREAKFAST

4 fl oz (100 ml) orange juice; 5 oz (125 g) low-fat natural yogurt mixed with ¹/₂ oz (12.5 g) oats, ¹/₂ oz (12.5 g) sultanas, 3 oz (75 g) sliced banana and 1 tsp honey

or

¹/₄ pint/5 fl oz (125 ml) orange juice; 1 slice very lean bacon, grilled, plus unlimited grilled tomatoes and mushrooms
1 oz (25 g) wholemeal toast (no butter)

LUNCH

Ⓟ Chicken and Sweetcorn Sandwich

2 slices (3 oz/75 g) wholemeal bread spread with reduced-oil salad dressing and filled with 2 oz (50 g) chopped chicken, 2 oz (50 g) sweetcorn, plus salad

Ⓠ Knickerbocker Glory

Take a tall stemmed glass and fill with alternate spoons of 6 oz (150 g) jelly, 2 oz (50 g) low-fat cottage cheese, 5 oz (125 g) diet yogurt and 4 oz (100 g) Wall's 'Too Good To Be True' ice cream plus 4 oz (100 g) chopped fresh fruit

Ⓡ American Turkey Burgers (page 160)

DINNER

STARTER
1 oz (25 g) Parma ham with fan of melon

Ⓡ Trout Parcels with Dill Sauce (page 168)

Ⓠ Chicken Provençale with Peppers and Onions (page 164)

Ⓥ Chickpea and Fennel Casserole (page 170)

DESSERT
Hot Cherries (page 177)

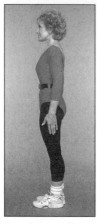 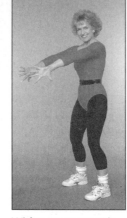 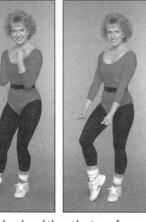 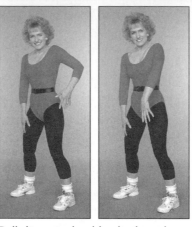 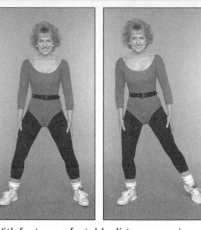

Start by standing tall, tummy in, shoulder blades back and down.

With your arms out in front, rotate arms inwards and outwards 8 times.

Tap the heel and then the toe of one foot, flexing and straightening both arms. Do 8, then repeat with the other foot.

Roll alternate shoulders backwards, transferring your weight from one foot to the other. Do 16, then repeat, rolling shoulders forwards.

With feet a comfortable distance apart, transfer your weight from one foot to the other, bending your knees and tapping the toes of the opposite foot as you step. Do 16.

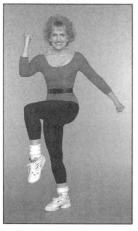 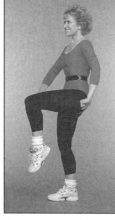 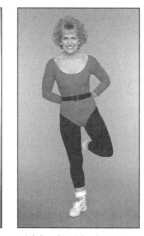 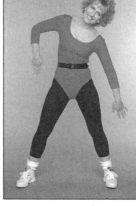 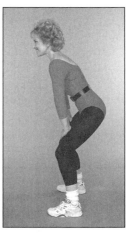

Raise alternate knees and aim to touch with opposite elbow. Do 16.

Raise alternate knees in front, pressing down with both arms. Keep your tummy tight and back straight. Do 16.

Extend alternate legs to the side, pointing your toes and swinging your arms in and out as you step. Do 16.

Kick back with alternate feet. Do 16.

With feet a comfortable distance apart, lean over to the side without twisting the hips. Repeat to the other side. Do 8 to each side.

With feet wide apart, bend your knees and go down into a squat, making sure the knees bend over the ankles. Come up again, and repeat. Do 8.

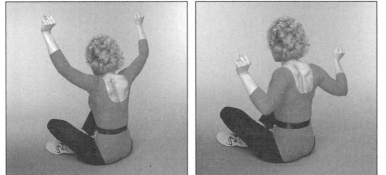

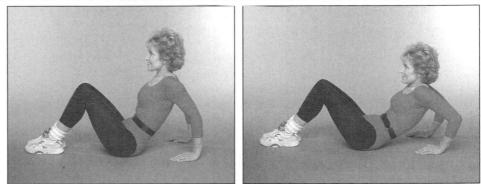

Upper Back Toner Sit upright with your legs crossed. Take your arms above your head and reach up. Now pull the elbows back and down to squeeze your shoulder blades together. Raise the arms again, and repeat. Do 14–16.

Upper Arm Toner Sit with knees bent and prop yourself up on your hands. Your hands should be placed at least 12 inches (30 cm) behind your back, with fingers pointing forwards. Bend your arms so that your elbows move backwards, then straighten them again. Do 10–12.

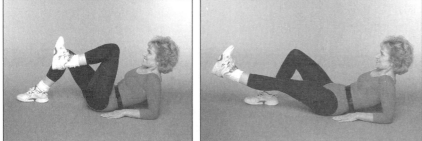

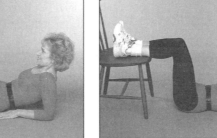

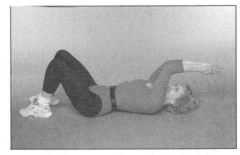

Front Thigh Toner Supporting yourself on your arms, bend both knees. Bring one knee in towards your chest and then extend the leg straight out in front. Keep your tummy tight to support your back. Bring the leg towards your chest again, and repeat. Do 12–14, then repeat with the other leg.

Tummy Toner Place your feet against a wall or on a sturdy chair, and support your head with your hands. *Pulling your tummy in tightly*, raise your head and shoulders off the floor, keeping a distance between your chin and your chest. Raise on a count of 2, and return to the floor on a count of 2. Repeat 14–16 times.

Chest Toner Lie on your back with knees bent and place your arms out to the sides with elbows bent at shoulder level. Lift your arms and press the elbows and palms together. Keeping the arms together and parallel with the floor, push them over your head and then pull them forwards again. Repeat this backwards and forwards movement 14–16 times, keeping the elbows together throughout the exercise.

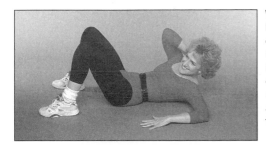

Waist Toner Place one hand behind your neck and have the other arm on the floor for support. Raise the head and shoulder and bring your elbow towards the opposite knee, taking care not to roll your hips. Return to the floor, and repeat. Do 14–16, then repeat to the other side.

CONTINUED ▶

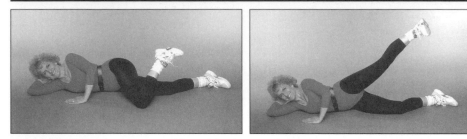

Outer Thigh Toner Lie on your side with both knees slightly bent. Dip the knee of the top leg on the floor in front and then, leading with the heel, extend and straighten it towards the corner of the room. Repeat this dipping and straightening movement 12–14 times, ensuring the hips remain square. Roll over, and repeat with the other leg.

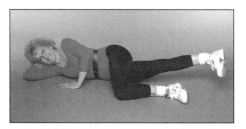

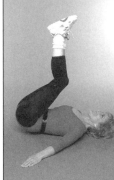

Inner Thigh Toner Bend the top leg and rest it on the floor in front of you. Keeping the bottom leg straight, lift it up and down 12–14 times. Roll over, and repeat with the other leg.

Tummy Trimmer Lying with legs raised and slightly bent, press your tummy muscles down and lift the hips slightly off the floor. Repeat 14–16 times, ensuring the effort comes from your abdomen, not your arms.

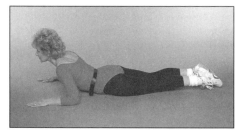

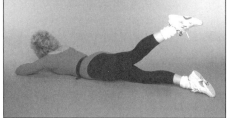

Back Strengthener Lie on your front and place your arms to the sides with elbows bent, palms facing upwards. Slowly raise your chest off the floor, using the muscles in your back not your arms. Return to the floor and repeat. Do 12–14.

Bottom Toner Resting your head on your hands, raise one leg straight up and down, squeezing your seat as you raise. Keep your hips pressed into the floor throughout. Do 12–14, then repeat with the other leg.

Tummy Stretch Place your arms out to the sides with elbows bent. Slowly raise your head and shoulders off the floor, supporting yourself on your forearms and elbows, and feel the stretch down the front of your abdomen. Hold for 10 seconds.

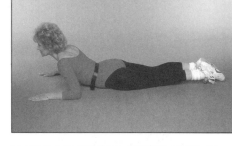

Front Thigh Stretch Resting your face on one hand, bend the opposite leg and use your hand to ease it towards your seat. Hold for 10 seconds then release, and repeat with the other leg.

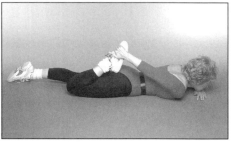

Back Stretch Position yourself on all fours and arch the spine as much as possible, pulling your tummy towards your spine. Hold for 10 seconds.

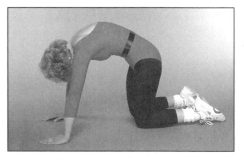

Seat Stretch Lie on your back with knees towards your chest, and place your hands underneath your thighs. Ease your legs further towards your chest and feel the stretch in your seat. Hold for 10 seconds.

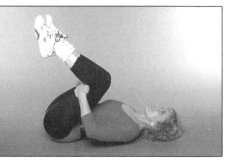

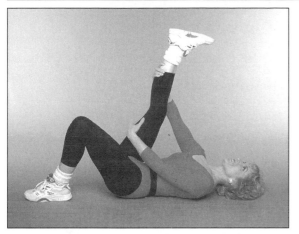

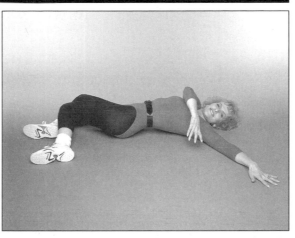

Back of Thigh Stretch Place both feet on the floor. Take hold of one leg and raise it, straightening it as far as is comfortable. Ease the leg towards you with your hands and hold for 10–15 seconds. Relax, and repeat with the other leg.

Waist and Outer Thigh Stretch Lying on your back with both knees bent, allow your knees to drop to one side while taking your arms to the opposite side. Hold for 10 seconds, then slowly return to the centre, and repeat to the other side.

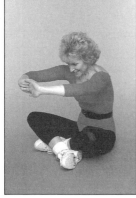

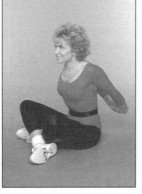

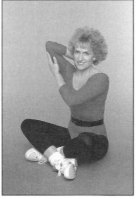

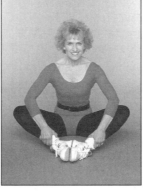

Upper Back Stretch Sitting with legs crossed, round your back and raise your arms in front to shoulder level to separate your shoulder blades. Hold for 10 seconds.

Chest Stretch Raise your arms and clasp your hands behind your back to stretch the muscles across your chest. Hold for 10 seconds.

Back of Upper Arm Stretch Raise one elbow and ease your hand down your back. Use the other arm to ease it further. Hold for 10 seconds. Repeat with the other arm.

Inner Thigh Stretch Sit up with knees bent and soles of the feet together. Using your elbows, gently ease your knees down as far as is comfortable. Hold for 15 seconds

You are now at the end of your second week and you must be feeling so much more confident. Keep building your confidence and register how much it is growing. Continue to make the best of yourself, learn to adopt good posture at all times, stand tall and enjoy the new you. Look forward to the next 14 days. Don't even question whether you are going to succeed. Just go for it. You will be ever so pleased that you did.

Yesterday we looked at the difference between a positive and a negative person, how a positive person can bring sunshine into your life whereas a negative one can make it cloudy and miserable all the time. There is nothing wrong with constructive criticism and, given with goodwill, this can help us enormously to get things right, to improve and to grow. But so little criticism is constructive and it is so easy to be destructive. We should think very carefully before we criticise others. Can we find a better way of doing things?

It's a good idea to check our own thoughts occasionally to see whether they are negative or positive. What are we honestly thinking? Are *we* being negative or positive? We should also build a bulletproof screen against people who are negative towards us. Negative comments can be very cutting and upsetting, but we have to learn to cope with them and not allow them to affect us too badly. As a friend once said to me, what other people say about you is none of your business. What a wise comment. It is one that I have taken on board and thought of many times.

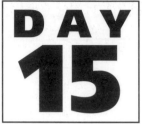

DAY 15

Well, isn't this great! Two weeks under your belt and your waist is significantly narrower. Pop on the scales, then measure yourself carefully and tot up the inches that you have lost. You probably will not have lost as much weight as the previous week but you should have lost inches. When the inches disappear it is a clear indication of the fat being burnt away. Don't be disheartened if the weight loss is not as great as you thought it would be. It's the inches that really count and it's a flatter stomach that we are aiming for.

Now that you are familiar with the diet and it all seems to be comparatively easy, do not fall into the trap of thinking you can make your own adjustments to the meals and enjoy the same results, although meals can be repeated from earlier days. All the meals contained in this programme are calorie counted and designed to give you maximum nutrition, minimum fat with the ultimate in palatability. Just eating low-fat foods is not sufficient to enable you to lose weight. Calories need to be carefully controlled and finely balanced so that you eat enough to enable your body to function at its optimum but at the same time encourage it to draw on its excesses of fat for the extra fuel it needs. Never be tempted to go on a crash diet or use meal replacement foods. If you are to enjoy any chance of long-term success it is crucial that you 're-educate' your shopping trolley, your refrigerator, your frying pan and your palate. Having a liquid meal substitute is a false way of dieting. All you will do in the end is to go back to the foods that made you fat in the first place. Unless you understand which foods *made* you overweight and decide not to eat those in the future, you will never make any real progress. If there is a particular food that you really enjoy and it isn't included in the diet, check the nutrition panel on the product. Providing the calories, the fat content and the nutritional benefits are similar to the food that you wish to exchange, there is no reason why you should not make a substitute. It will take care and attention but if you are determined to do so, you can make it work.

Enjoy yourself today. Feel slim, stand tall and remember your posture. Keep your willpower as strong as ever and realise that, having crossed the halfway mark, you are now on the homeward straight. Well done, and keep going!

MENU

BREAKFAST

¹/₄ pint/5 fl oz (125 ml) orange juice; 1 oz (25 g) Special K and 10 sultanas mixed with 5 oz (125 g) low-fat natural yogurt and 1 tsp demerara sugar

or

¹/₄ pint/5 fl oz (125 ml) orange juice; 4 brown Ryvitas spread with 1 tsp marmalade; 1 x 5 oz (125 g) diet yogurt

LUNCH

℗ Tuna and Salad Pitta
1 wholemeal pitta filled with 2 oz (50 g) tuna (in brine), low-fat coleslaw, shredded lettuce, sliced tomato, cucumber, onion, pepper 1 x 5 oz (125 g) diet yogurt

Ⓞ Jacket Potato with Tuna
8 oz (200 g) jacket potato topped with 4 oz (100 g) tuna (in brine) mixed with 1 tbsp reduced-oil salad dressing, plus mixed salad

Ⓡ Haricot Bean and Vegetable Soup (page 159)
plus 1 slice wholemeal bread (no butter)

DINNER

STARTER
Water Melon with Mint Yogurt Sauce
6 oz (150 g) water melon finely chopped and mixed with 3 oz (75 g) low-fat natural yogurt and 1 tsp mint sauce

Ⓡ Chilli Chicken (page 165)

Ⓞ Sweet and Sour Chicken or Prawns with Crispy Vegetables (page 166)

Ⓥ Quorn Bolognese (page 171)

DESSERT
Prunes with Fromage Frais
Soak 4 prunes in tea overnight and serve with 2 tsp low-fat fromage frais

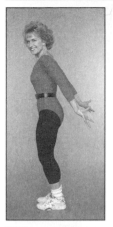

With your arms behind your back, rotate arms inwards and outwards. Do 8.

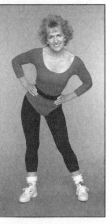

Take two steps to the side, swinging arms in and out as you step. Repeat to the other side. Do 16 to alternate sides.

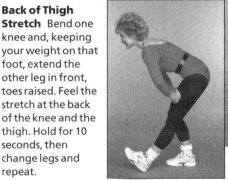

Rotate your hips in a clockwise direction. Do 8, then repeat in an anti-clockwise direction.

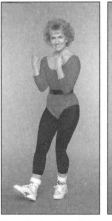
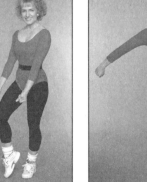

Tap the heel and then the toe of one foot, flexing and straightening both arms. Do 8, then repeat with the other foot.

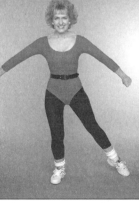

Extend alternate legs to the side, pointing your toes and swinging your arms in and out as you step. Do 16.

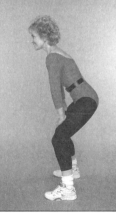

With feet wide apart, bend your knees and go down into a squat, making sure the knees bend over the ankles. Come up again, and repeat. Do 8.

Chest Stretch Take your arms behind you and place one hand on top of the other. Raise your arms and feel the stretch across your chest. Hold for 10 seconds.

Back of Thigh Stretch Bend one knee and, keeping your weight on that foot, extend the other leg in front, toes raised. Feel the stretch at the back of the knee and the thigh. Hold for 10 seconds, then change legs and repeat.

Calf Stretch Shift your weight on to the front leg and bend the knee. Your back leg is straight, heel on the floor and toes of both feet facing straight ahead. Keep your weight slightly forwards and feel the stretch in the calf muscle of your back leg. Hold for 10 seconds, then change legs and repeat.

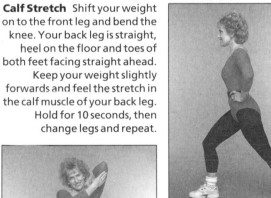

Back of Upper Arm Stretch Stand with feet a comfortable distance apart and knees slightly bent. Raise one elbow and ease your hand down your back, using the other arm to assist. Hold for 10 seconds. Relax, and repeat with the other arm.

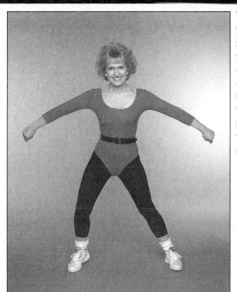

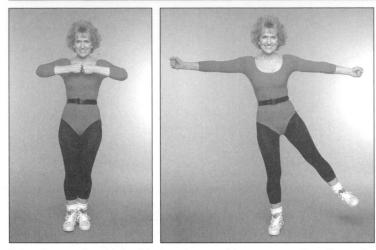

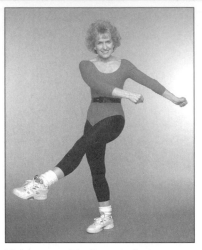

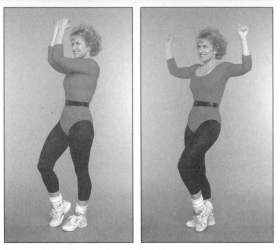

Raise alternate legs to the side, keeping your hips square and bending and straightening your arms at shoulder level. Do 24.

Kick across with alternate feet, swinging your arms from side to side. Do 32.

Do a walking jog on the spot, taking your bent arms in and out at shoulder level. Do 24.

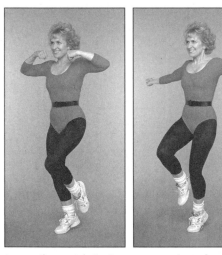

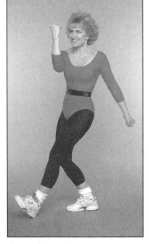

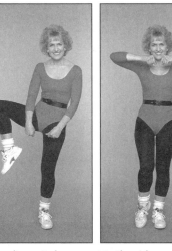

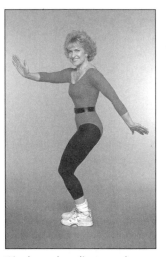

Jog on the spot, bringing your arms in and out at shoulder level. Do 32.

Swing one elbow across as you tap the opposite heel in front. Repeat with the other elbow and heel. Do 24 to alternate sides.

Raise alternate knees out to the side, pushing your arms down and up in 'barrow boy' style as you step. Do 32.

Dip down, bending your knees and reaching across with alternate arms. Do 32.

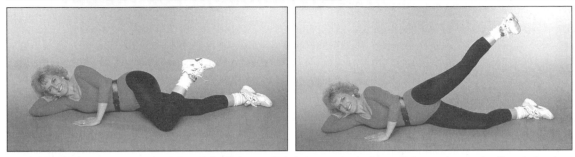

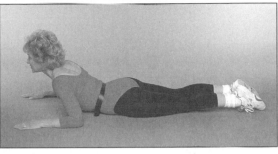

Outer Thigh Toner Lie on your side with both knees slightly bent. Dip the knee of the top leg on the floor in front and then, leading with the heel, extend and straighten it towards the corner of the room. Repeat this dipping and straightening movement 12–14 times, ensuring the hips remain square. Roll over, and repeat with the other leg.

Back Strengthener Lie face down with arms bent, palms facing upwards. Slowly raise your chest off the floor, using the muscles in your back not your arms. Return to the floor and repeat. Do 8–10.

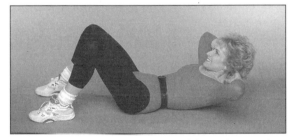

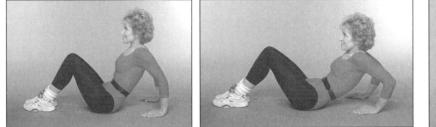

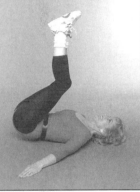

Tummy Toner Lie on your back with knees bent and your *tummy pulled in tightly*. Place your hands behind your neck and slowly raise your head and shoulders off the floor. Raise on a count of 2, then return to the floor on a count of 2, keeping a distance between your chin and your chest. Breathe out as you raise and breathe in as you go down. Do 14–16.

Upper Arm Toner Sit with knees bent and prop yourself up on your hands. Your hands should be placed at least 12 inches (30 cm) behind your back, with fingers pointing forwards. Bend your arms so that your elbows move backwards, then straighten them again. Do 10–12.

Tummy Trimmer Lie on your back with legs raised and slightly bent. Your feet are over your hips and your tummy is pulled in tightly. Press your tummy muscles down and lift the hips slightly off the floor. Repeat 14–16 times, ensuring the effort comes from your abdomen, not your arms.

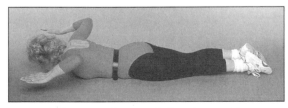

Inner Thigh Toner With legs raised directly above your hips and soles of the feet aiming towards the ceiling, allow the legs to separate, then bring them together again. Keep your back pressed into the floor throughout. Do 14–16.

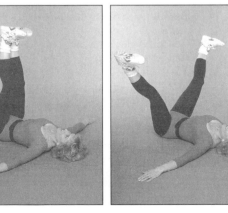

Upper Back Strengthener Lie face down with arms bent at shoulder level. Raise your arms, squeezing your shoulder blades together as much as possible, then lower your arms. Repeat 12–14 times.

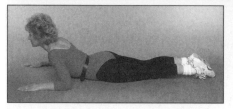

Tummy Stretch Lie face down with arms bent. Slowly raise your head and shoulders off the floor, supporting yourself on your forearms and elbows, and feel the stretch down the front of your abdomen. Hold for 10 seconds.

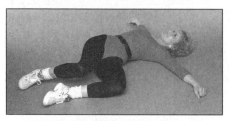

Outer Thigh Stretch Lying with arms outstretched and knees bent, lower both knees slowly to one side, keeping both feet on the floor. Hold for 10 seconds. Slowly raise the knees to the centre, and repeat to the other side.

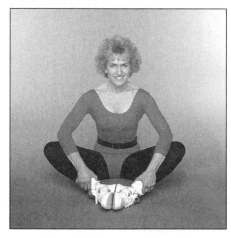

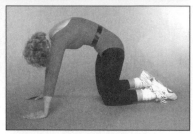

Back Stretch Position yourself on all fours and arch the spine as much as possible, pulling your tummy towards your spine. Hold for 10 seconds.

Upper Back Stretch Round your back and raise your arms in front to shoulder level to separate your shoulder blades. Hold for 10 seconds.

Inner Thigh Stretch Sit up with knees bent and soles of the feet together. Using your elbows, gently ease your knees down as far as is comfortable. Hold for 15 seconds.

POSITIVE THOUGHT FOR THE DAY

Here we are on the first day of the third week. You have followed the diet and exercises for 14 days and you should be feeling stronger and fitter. You will have effectively burnt some fat from your body so that you are now physically trimmer. The inches and the pounds are disappearing, and you should be delighted with the progress you have made. You have achieved the first half of your first goal – a goal that required a great deal of determination and a huge amount of effort on your part. When you reach the end of the 28-day period you will be so pleased with your results that there will be no holding you from then on. Your posture will have improved, your eating habits will have changed for the better and your energy level will have greatly increased. I am sure your family will be happier too. You are now realising that having a goal and working towards it really does pay dividends.

So many people blame lack of time as the reason for not achieving their hopes and dreams. Your aim may be to attend a night-school class to learn a second language or a particular craft. Or it may be simply to spend more time with your family or to be able to cope better with a job, whether full or part-time. If we manage our time well, we can achieve so much more.

Over the last few years my life has changed dramatically and the demands on my time have become ever greater. I believe I achieve a lot because I 'manage' my time carefully and use it to the full. I rarely work at weekends, which allows Mike and me to spend quality time together and to recharge our batteries. After all, why work so hard if you don't have time to enjoy your leisure? At any one time I have several projects in the pipeline whether it be a book, a video or a TV series. Each project is given quality time that is allocated in advance and I allow nothing to interrupt those plans. The vast amount of correspondence I receive is dealt with during car journeys if I am being driven, or on the train, or in between appointments. I do not spend time worrying about a project before it is necessary to do so, but rather spend time finishing the current one. It is vital that we get our priorities right and concentrate on the most important tasks to be done.

Finding time to exercise each day is very important too. I tend to go for a run with the dogs at six in the morning as this starts me off for the day in fine form. There is little traffic about at that time and I am able to enjoy the countryside at its best. For the first few mornings it was tough but now I look forward to it and it has become a habit which I really miss if it's raining (I'm a fair weather jogger!). The feeling of satisfaction when we have done our exercises is terrific and well worth the effort.

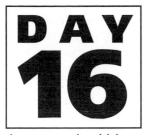

DAY 16

As we progress into the third week let us take a closer look at fat in our diet. Fat is a high-energy food because it is high in calories. Since we can get all the energy we need from carbohydrates, we should keep fat to an absolute minimum. Unless you are an infant or an élite athlete, the fat you eat turns to fat on the body – you just don't need it. In a varied diet we will obtain sufficient fat to stay healthy without the need to use butter, spreads, fats or oils in our food preparation. What we *do* need is lots of carbohydrates such as potatoes, bread, rice, pasta and cereal. These form a vital part of our daily diet as they are energy-giving foods which will be used efficiently by the body and will not turn to fat unless taken in excess. Remember, if we eat too much of *anything* we will store the excess as fat. Over a period of months or years of bad eating habits those pounds can creep up on us. The diet contained in this book includes sufficient fat for health. However, vegetarians will need to use a little extra fat in their food preparation, since they will not be benefiting from the fat that is contained in meat, poultry and fish. I have taken this into account in the vegetarian recipes in this book.

Many of us acquired the habit of eating fat from our parents, as they did from their parents. But we now live in an age where there are so many labour-saving devices that the level of physical activity necessary for survival is dramatically reduced. We have to make a concerted effort to get fitter, whereas years ago it happened automatically. But bad habits can be exchanged for good ones, so stop using lard or oil for cooking and make physical activity part of your daily routine. Enjoy your day.

MENU

BREAKFAST

4 fl oz (100 ml) orange juice; 2 bananas mashed or sliced with 5 oz (125 g) diet yogurt and ¹/₂ oz (12.5 g) sultanas

or

¹/₄ pint/5 fl oz (125 ml) orange juice; ³/₄ oz (18.5) All-Bran and ³/₄ oz (18.5 g) cornflakes, served with 4 fl oz (100 ml) milk in addition to allowance and 2 tsp demerara sugar

LUNCH

P 4 brown Ryvitas spread with Branston pickle and topped with 3 oz (75 g) chicken, turkey or ham, plus salad

Q 2 slices wholemeal light bread topped with 6 oz (150 g) baked beans; 1 piece fresh fruit

R *Jacket Potato and Stir-fry Vegetables*
8 oz (200 g) jacket potato topped with 6 oz (150 g) cooked stir-fry vegetables (frozen ready prepared)
1 x 5 oz (125 g) low-fat fromage frais (fruit variety) or diet fruit yogurt

DINNER

STARTER
¹/₂ fresh grapefruit

R *Campfire Kidneys* (page 161)

Q *Chinese Chicken with Pineapple* (page 165)

V *Vegetable Chop Suey* (page 173)

DESSERT
Kiwi Fruit Sorbet (page 177)

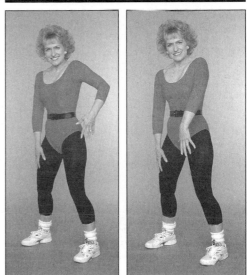

Roll alternate shoulders backwards, transferring your weight from one foot to the other. Do 16, then repeat, rolling shoulders forwards.

Step from side to side and tap the opposite heel on the floor in front, flexing and straightening your arms as you step. Do 16.

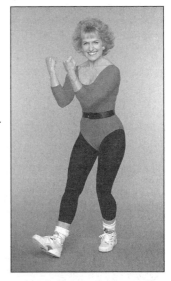

CONTINUED ▶

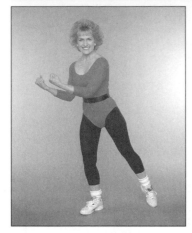

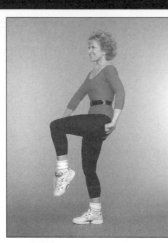

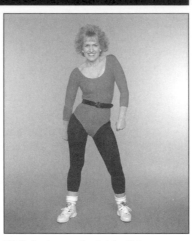

Take two steps to the side, making a scooping movement with your arms as if shovelling snow. Repeat to the other side. Do 16, alternating sides.

Raise alternate knees in front, pressing down with both arms. Keep your tummy tight and back straight. Do 16.

With feet a comfortable distance apart, raise one hip and at the same time raise the opposite shoulder. Repeat with the other hip and shoulder. Do 16 on alternate sides.

Back of Thigh Stretch Bend one knee and, keeping your weight on that foot, extend the other leg in front, toes raised. Feel the stretch at the back of the knee and the thigh. Hold for 10 seconds, then change legs and repeat.

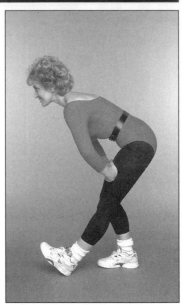

With one arm raised, palm facing upwards, and the other hand on your hip, lean directly to the side, reaching over with the raised arm. Do not twist the hips. Return to the starting position and repeat to the other side. Do 8 to each side.

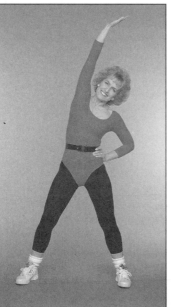

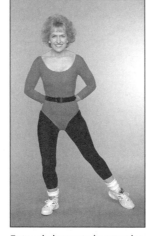

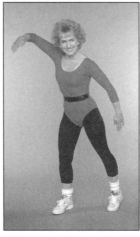

Extend alternate legs to the side, tapping the toes to the floor as you step. Do 16.

Circle alternate arms in a front crawl swimming motion, transferring your weight from one foot to the other. Do 16.

Calf Stretch Shift your weight on to the front leg and bend the knee. Your back leg is straight, heel on the floor and toes of both feet facing straight ahead. Keep your weight slightly forwards and feel the stretch in the calf muscle of your back leg. Hold for 10 seconds, then change legs and repeat.

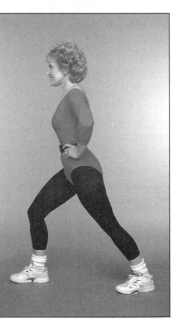

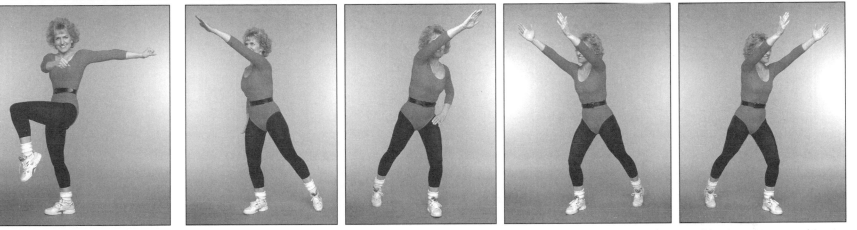

Keeping your tummy pulled in throughout, raise alternate knees across your body, swinging your arms from side to side. Do 24.

Reach across with one arm and tap the opposite foot to the floor in a diagonal position. Do 24 to alternate sides then repeat, reaching both arms across.

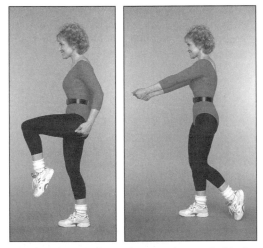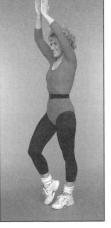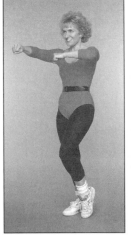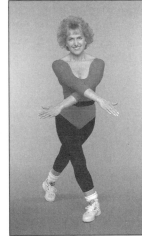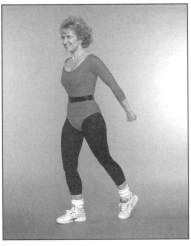

Raise one knee in front, then tap the toes behind, bringing the arms backwards and forwards as if pulling drawers out and in. Keep your tummy tight throughout. Do 32, then repeat with the other leg.

March on the spot, clapping your hands above your head. Do 24.

March on the spot and punch alternate hands forwards. Don't stamp. Do 32.

Step to the side and curtsey with one leg behind, swinging your arms out to the side then crossing them in front as you step. Do 32.

Tap the toes of alternate feet on the floor behind, pushing your arms back as you tap. Do 32.

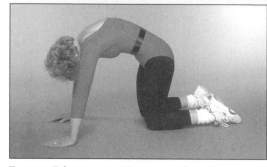

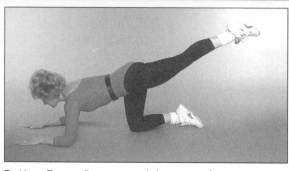

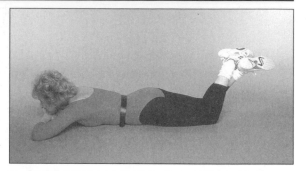

Tummy Trimmer Position yourself on all fours and pull your tummy muscles in as tightly as you can to arch your spine. Relax, and repeat 14–16 times.

Bottom Toner Rest your weight on your forearms. Extend one leg behind you. Keeping the leg straight, raise it in line with your hips – no higher – then lower it again. Raise and lower the leg 12–14 times, keeping your tummy in and your back flat throughout. Repeat with the other leg.

Back of Thigh Toner Lie face down with your head resting on your hands, and cross your ankles. Bend your knees and slowly raise your ankles off the floor, using the resistance of the top leg to make the exercise more difficult. Lower the ankles, and repeat. Do 10–12, then repeat with the other ankle on top.

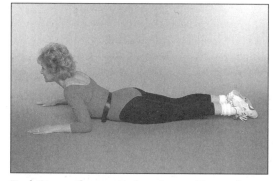

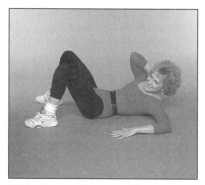

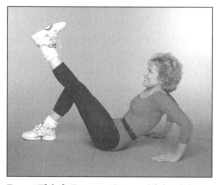

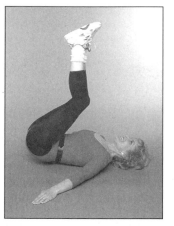

Back Strengthener Lie face down with arms bent, palms facing upwards. Slowly raise your chest off the floor, using the muscles in your back not your arms. Return to the floor and repeat. Do 14–16.

Waist Toner Lie on your back with knees bent. Place one hand behind your neck and have the other arm on the floor for support. Raise the head and shoulder and bring your elbow towards the opposite knee, taking care not to roll your hips. Return to the floor, and repeat. Do 14–16, then repeat to the other side.

Front Thigh Toner Sit up with both legs bent, and support your weight on your hands. Straighten one leg and raise it to the level of the other knee, then lower it again. Do 12–14 straight leg lifts, keeping your tummy tight. Repeat with the other leg.

Tummy Trimmer Lie on your back with legs raised and slightly bent. Your feet are over your hips and your tummy is pulled in tightly. Press your tummy muscles down and lift the hips slightly off the floor. Repeat 14–16 times, ensuring the effort comes from your abdomen, not your arms.

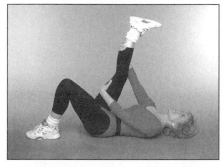

Back of Thigh Stretch Place both feet on the floor. Take hold of one leg and raise it, straightening it as far as is comfortable. Ease the leg towards you with your hands and hold for 10–15 seconds. Relax, and repeat with the other leg.

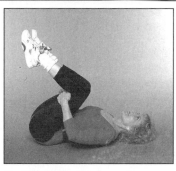

Seat Stretch Bend your knees towards your chest and place your hands underneath your thighs. Ease your legs further towards your chest and feel the stretch in your seat. Hold for 10 seconds.

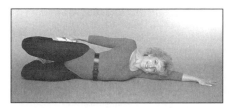

Front Thigh Stretch Lie on your side with both legs bent. Keeping the hips square, ease the foot of the top leg back, using your hand to assist. Hold for 10 seconds. Roll over and repeat with the other leg.

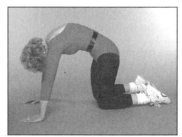

Back Stretch Position yourself on all fours and arch the spine as much as possible, pulling the tummy towards the spine. Hold for 10 seconds.

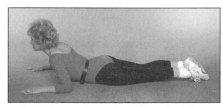

Tummy Stretch Lie face down with arms bent. Slowly raise your head and shoulders off the floor, supporting yourself on your forearms and elbows, and feel the stretch down the front of your abdomen. Hold for 10 seconds.

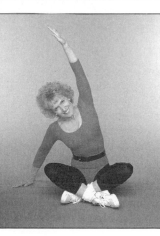

Waist Stretch Sit up with legs crossed. Place one hand on the floor for support, and reach over to the side with the other arm. Hold for 10 seconds, then relax and repeat to the other side.

POSITIVE THOUGHT FOR THE DAY

You must be feeling delighted with your progress so far and I hope this feeling of well-being will encourage you to continue. Take particular note of how many more repetitions you are able to do of the various toning exercises, how much fitter you are and the length of time for which you arc able to continue in the aerobic section. If you wish, you can repeat the toning exercises so that you complete the sequence and then do another set of each.

Exercise needs to be sustained, and once you have completed this programme you may wish to use the Flat Stomach Plan workout video (see end of book for details) to maintain your new shape. There are also Rosemary Conley Diet and Fitness Clubs throughout the UK which are most welcoming to anyone who cares to join. The exercises are taught by qualified instructors, all of whom have been personally selected by me. If you feel that you require weekly support and friendship, you will find it in abundance at these classes (see end of book for details). Again it comes down to scoring goals. Each member who comes along to one of our classes goes away with a one-week challenge to be as good as possible before their weighing session the following week. A dieter can easily cope with these short-term goals and this is why it works so superbly.

Remember we need to push positive thinking all the way in all areas of our life – personal and professional. You can't be negative about parts of your life and positive about others. Always bear in mind that your chances of motivating people to do what you want are much greater if you are positive. If you want your family to change some habits you need to make them realise the benefits. If by helping out with the daily chores they discover that you now have time for a family picnic, to go swimming or go to the zoo, they will soon realise the benefit of pulling together. Sell the idea to them! *We* hold the controls, and all it takes is a little thought to put a request in a positive way. Remember, people going nowhere normally get there, but people who have goals are those that achieve.

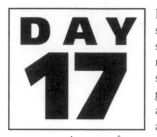

DAY 17

By now you should be feeling significantly trimmer and fitter. We should look at a good low-fat diet as our passport to a leaner body, and treat exercise as a fun way to achieve a full and healthy life. Thankfully, gone are the days of calorie counting and weighing everything we ate. That was so boring.

Today's exercises are more challenging, and the more challenging the activity the more benefit we are likely to enjoy. If we were to continue to do exactly the same exercises without progressing, the benefits would diminish. We can only increase our level of fitness by placing greater demands on the body. Don't worry, I'm not going to ask you to start training for a marathon. I certainly would not recommend that to anyone but the most dedicated. We don't need to exercise at that level to enjoy 100 per cent fitness. Playing sport or keeping fit in many different ways can be much more fun than sitting watching television. And spending time in the open air is infinitely healthier than breathing in smoke in a stuffy bar! As you will have learned over the last two and a half weeks, if we combine increased physical activity with a good healthy low-fat diet, our energy levels increase quite measurably.

Enjoy today's menus, perform the exercises precisely and do as many repetitions as you can without feeling too tired. Continue to maintain a good posture, paying particular attention to your abdominal area. Have a great day.

MENU

BREAKFAST

¹/₄ pint/5 fl oz (125 ml) orange juice; 1¹/₂ oz (37.5 g) porridge oats cooked in water and left overnight, served with 3 fl oz (75 ml) milk (in addition to allowance) plus 2 tsp honey

or

Orange and Grapefruit Cocktail

(page 157) plus 1 slice wholemeal toast spread with 1 tsp marmalade

LUNCH

P 1 wholemeal bread roll (2 oz/50 g) filled with salad and low-fat coleslaw; 1 x 8 oz (200 g) pot Müllerlight yogurt

Q 2 slices (3 oz/75 g) wholemeal toast topped with 8 oz (200 g) canned tomatoes boiled well and reduced to a creamy consistency and 4 oz (100 g) baked beans; 1 piece fresh fruit

R *Jacket Potato with Curried Chicken and Yogurt Topping* (page 160)

DINNER

STARTER
Marinated Haddock (page 157)

R **Chicken Paprika** (page 164)

Q **Jalfrezi Chicken Curry with Rice**
Allow 6 oz (150 g) chicken breast per person. Chop and dry-fry in a non-stick pan. When nearly cooked add 16 oz (400 g) Patak's Original Jalfrezi Cooking Sauce (serves 4) and continue cooking for 10 minutes. Serve with boiled brown rice (2 oz/50 g [dry weight] per person)

V **Mixed Bean Hotpot** (page 171)

DESSERT
1 piece fresh fruit plus 1 x 5 oz (125 g) diet yogurt

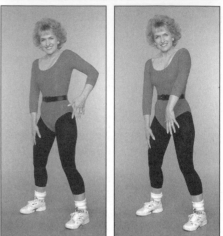

Roll alternate shoulders backwards, transferring your weight from one foot to the other. Do 16, then repeat, rolling shoulders forwards.

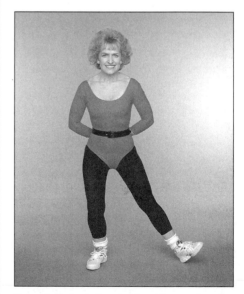

Extend alternate legs to the side, tapping the floor with your heels. Do 16

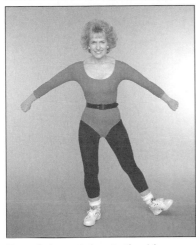

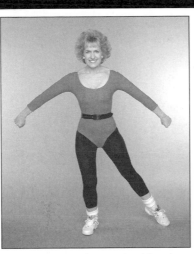

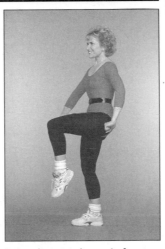

Extend alternate legs to the side, tapping the floor with your heels and swinging your arms in and out. Do 16.

Extend alternate legs to the side, pointing your toes and swinging your arms in and out. Do 16.

Raise alternate knees in front, pressing down with both arms. Keep your tummy tight and back straight. Do 16.

Back of Thigh Stretch Bend one knee and, keeping your weight on that foot, extend the other leg in front, toes raised. Feel the stretch at the back of the knee and the thigh. Hold for 10 seconds, then change legs and repeat.

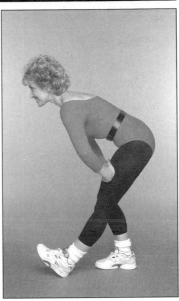

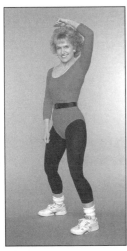

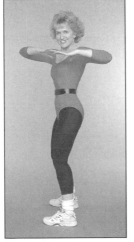

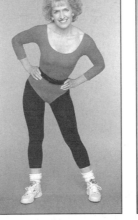

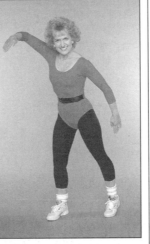

Rotate alternate arms backwards as if brushing your hair, transferring your weight from one foot to the other. Do 16.

Keeping your hips square, twist your upper body from side to side. Do not jerk. Do 8 to each side.

Rotate your hips in a clockwise direction. Do 8, then repeat in an anti-clockwise direction.

Circle alternate arms in a front crawl swimming motion, transferring your weight from one foot to the other. Do 16.

Calf Stretch Shift your weight on to the front leg and bend the knee. Your back leg is straight, heel on the floor and toes of both feet facing straight ahead. Keep your weight slightly forwards and feel the stretch in the calf muscle of your back leg. Hold for 10 seconds, then change legs and repeat.

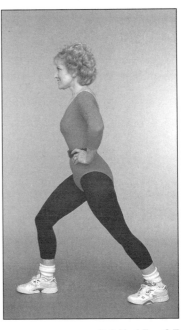

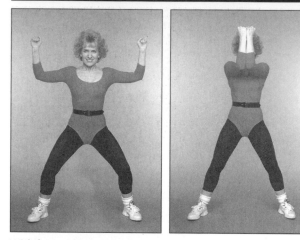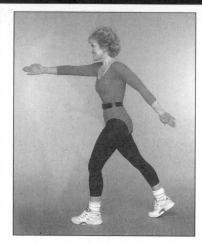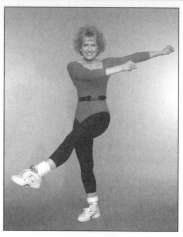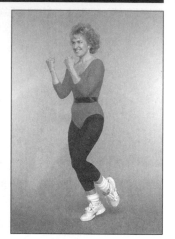

With feet wide apart and toes and knees facing slightly outwards, squat down, then come up again, bringing both arms out and in at shoulder level. Do 24.

Touch the floor behind with one foot and swing the same arm forwards. Bring the foot back to the centre and repeat with the other leg and arm. Do 24 on alternate sides.

Kick across with alternate feet, swinging your arms from side to side in the opposite direction to your feet. Do 32.

Jog on the spot, flexing and straightening both arms. Keep your knees soft and bring the heels down as you land. Do 32.

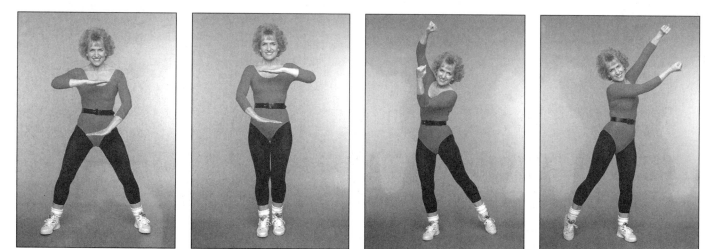

Take 2 steps to the side, pressing down with your hands as you step. Repeat to the other side. Do 32 to alternate sides.

Step and touch alternate feet to the floor, swinging your arms in a figure of eight as you step. Do 32.

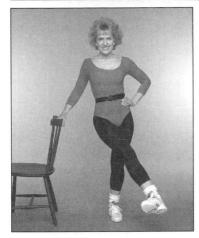

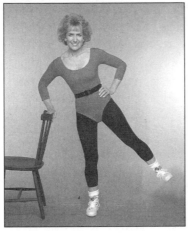

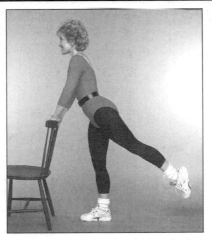

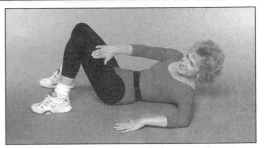

Waist Toner Lie on the floor with knees bent. Supporting yourself with one arm, reach across your body with the other arm, pressing your tummy down as you reach. Take care not to roll the hips. Return to the floor, and repeat. Do 16–18, then repeat to the other side.

Inner Thigh Toner Holding on to a chair, extend the inside leg forwards and across the body then back again. Keep your hips square. Do 14–16, then turn round and repeat with the other leg.

Outer Thigh Toner Raise the outside leg out to the side, keeping your hips square and toes pointing forwards. Lower the leg, and repeat. Do 14–16, then turn round and repeat with the other leg.

Bottom Toner Face the chair and raise one leg behind you, keeping the leg straight and squeezing your seat as you raise. Lower the leg, and repeat. Keep your tummy tight, hips square and your back straight throughout. Do 14–16, then repeat with the other leg.

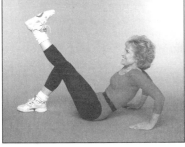

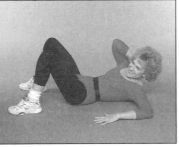

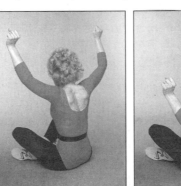

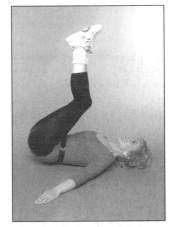

Front Thigh Toner Sit up with both legs bent, and support your weight on your hands. Straighten one leg and raise it to the level of the other knee, then lower it again. Do 12–14 straight leg lifts, keeping your tummy tight. Repeat with the other leg.

Waist Trimmer Lying on your back with both knees bent, place one hand behind your neck and have the other arm on the floor for support. Raise your head and shoulder and bring your elbow towards the opposite knee, taking care not to roll your hips. Return to the floor, and repeat. Do 16–18, then repeat to the other side.

Upper Back Toner Sit upright with your legs crossed. Take your arms above your head and reach up. Now pull the elbows back and down to squeeze your shoulder blades together. Raise the arms again, and repeat. Do 12–14.

Tummy Trimmer Lying on your back with legs raised and slightly bent, press your tummy muscles down and lift your hips slightly off the floor. Repeat 12–14 times, ensuring the effort comes from your abdomen, not your arms.

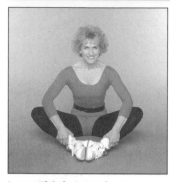

Inner Thigh Stretch Sit up with knees bent and soles of the feet together. Using your elbows, gently ease your knees down as far as is comfortable. Hold for 15 seconds.

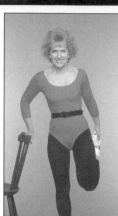

Front Thigh Stretch Stand and hold on to the back of a chair. Keeping your inside leg slightly bent, bend the other leg and take hold of your foot. Ease the foot back and up, keeping both knees aligned. Hold for 10 seconds. Release, then turn round and repeat with the other leg.

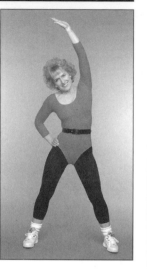

Waist Stretch Standing with feet a comfortable distance apart and knees slightly bent, place one hand on your thigh for support and lean to the side as you reach the opposite arm over. Hold for 10 seconds. Slowly straighten up, and repeat to the other side.

Full Body Stretch Standing upright, reach your arms towards the ceiling and hold for 10 seconds.

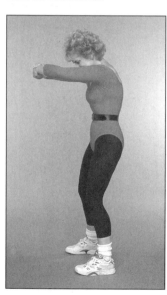

Upper Back Stretch Round your back and raise your arms in front to shoulder level to separate your shoulder blades. Hold for 10 seconds.

POSITIVE THOUGHT FOR THE DAY

I find music both enjoyable and motivational. In the case of exercise, music that is bright and cheerful makes you want to do it all the more and you will find you are able to continue for longer. So do play your favourite tracks or melodies to add extra enjoyment to your workout. Ideally, try to find a time or place to practise the routines where you won't be disturbed by the rest of the family. The more you are able to concentrate on the exercises, the better you will perform them and the greater the benefits.

Now, having motivated ourselves, let's look at how we can help others gain confidence, particularly the family members. It's really important to 'build up' your family. It's easy to get into the habit of putting your partner or children down. Millions of people do it without being aware of the fact. Often it's a reaction aimed at keeping the other person under control. But these put-downs can damage a family in the same way that knocking bricks out of a wall damages a building. Ask yourself if you ever put down someone in your family or do you build them up? Consider your answer carefully. Can you make any improvements? By changing *your* attitude you can set an example to the rest of the family. Start being generous with praise and try to keep the put-downs to an absolute minimum. Using the put-down policy tends to encourage the person who is being put down to look for the chinks in your armour so that they can then score one on you. It's amazing how complimenting people and learning to accept compliments can really produce a much more positive and happy environment for all concerned. Try and make a definite effort today to start decreasing the put-downs and increasing the praise. Watch the results. You'll be pleasantly surprised.

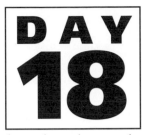

DAY 18

Eating a variety of foods that are low in fat but high in nutrition will provide the good quality nutrients we need to keep the body in good repair and enable it to perform the tasks we ask of it. It is important to understand what the food we eat actually does for us. Meat, fish, eggs and cheese are high-protein foods which help growth and repair. We don't need loads of protein – in fact too much can be harmful – and we need to select the protein that is low in fat such as lean meat, fish, poultry without skin, and low-fat cheese such as cottage cheese. Eggs should be restricted to just a couple a week as the yolk is high in fat.

We need vitamins and minerals to keep us healthy too and we can get a good supply if we eat fresh fruit and vegetables, low-fat dairy products and a good variety of foods generally. Fibre adds bulk to a diet, yet is low in calories, so always choose wholemeal alternatives where possible in order to take in more fibre. Calcium is very important particularly for middle-aged women because of their increased risk of osteoporosis. While milk is perhaps the best-known source of calcium, skimmed or semi-skimmed milk actually contains *more* calcium than the full-cream sort. However, children under five should always have full-cream milk because of the extra fat content but after five, semi-skimmed is fine. Dark green vegetables such as spinach and broccoli are also a rich source of calcium. Carbohydrates provide energy and can be found in potatoes, rice, pasta, cereals, fruit and vegetables. All the menus in this book are designed to contain a good variety of nutrients, so enjoy the menus today and select dishes that really whet your appetite.

MENU

BREAKFAST

4 fl oz (100 ml) orange juice; 2 slices light bread toasted or 1 slice wholemeal regular toast, topped with 4 oz (100 g) canned tomatoes boiled to reduce to a creamy consistency and 4 oz (100 g) baked beans
1 x 5 oz (125 g) diet yogurt

or

1/4 pint/5 fl oz (125 ml) orange juice;
2 Weetabix biscuits with 4 fl oz (100 ml) milk (in addition to allowance) and 2 tsp sugar

LUNCH

Ⓟ 4 brown Ryvitas spread with horseradish sauce and topped with 2 oz (50 g) wafer-thin beef, sliced beetroot and salad

Ⓠ 1 Heinz 'Lunchbowl' Chicken Curry with Rice; 1 piece fresh fruit

Ⓡ **Potato and Watercress Soup**
(page 159), plus 1 slice wholemeal bread or toast (no butter)

DINNER

STARTER
French Tomatoes (page156)

Ⓡ **Chicken Risotto** (page 165)

Ⓠ Findus Lean Cuisine Glazed Chicken with Rice

Ⓥ **Vegetable and Fruit Curry**
(page 172)

DESSERT
Fruit Brûlée (page 176)

With your arms out in front, rotate arms inwards and outwards 8 times.

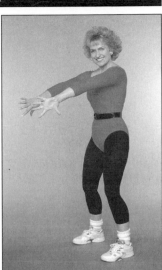

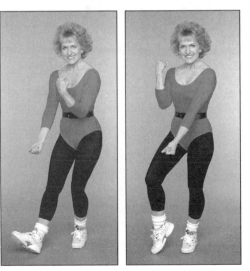

Tap the heel and then the toe of one foot, flexing and straightening alternate arms. Do 8, then repeat with the other foot.

CONTINUED ▶

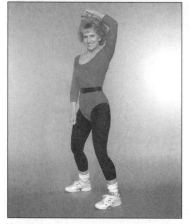

Rotate alternate arms backwards as if brushing your hair, transferring your weight from one foot to the other. Do 16.

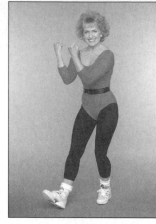

Step from side to side and tap alternate heels on the floor in front, flexing and straightening your arms as you step. Do 16.

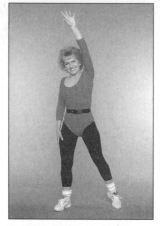

Transferring your weight from one foot to the other, swing alternate arms in complete circles. Do 16.

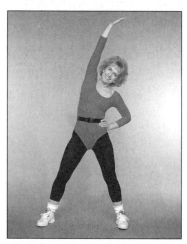

With one arm raised, palm facing upwards, and the other hand on your hip, lean directly to the side, reaching over with the raised arm. Do not twist the hips. Return to the starting position, and repeat to the other side. Do 8 to each side.

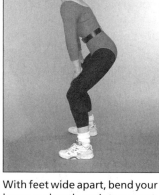

With feet wide apart, bend your knees and go down into a squat, making sure the knees bend over the ankles. Come up again, and repeat. Do 8.

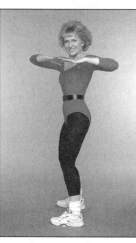

Keeping the hips square, twist your upper body from side to side. Do not jerk. Do 8 to each side.

Back of Thigh Stretch Bend one knee and, keeping your weight on that foot, extend the other leg in front, toes raised. Feel the stretch at the back of the knee and the thigh. Hold for 10 seconds, then change legs and repeat.

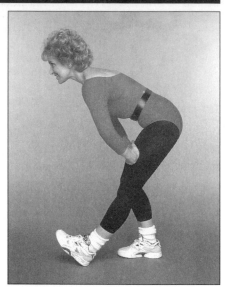

Calf Stretch Shift your weight on to the front leg and bend the knee. Your back leg is straight, heel on the floor and toes of both feet facing straight ahead. Keep your weight slightly forwards and feel the stretch in the calf muscle of your back leg. Hold for 10 seconds, then change legs and repeat.

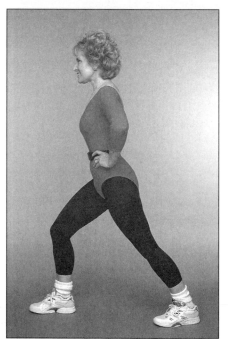

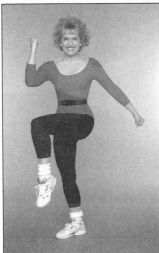

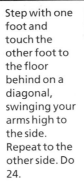

Step with one foot and touch the other foot to the floor behind on a diagonal, swinging your arms high to the side. Repeat to the other side. Do 24.

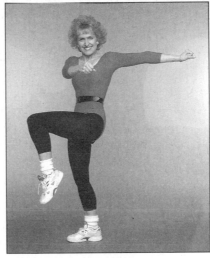

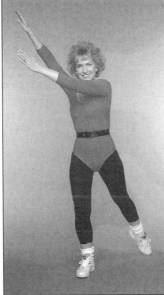

Raise alternate knees and aim to touch with opposite elbow. Do 16.

Keeping your tummy pulled in throughout, raise alternate knees across your body, swinging your arms from side to side. Do 24.

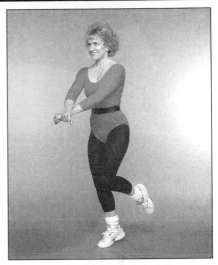

Jog on the spot, swinging your arms out and in and crossing them in front as you jog. Make sure the knees are soft and heels are down as you land. Do 32.

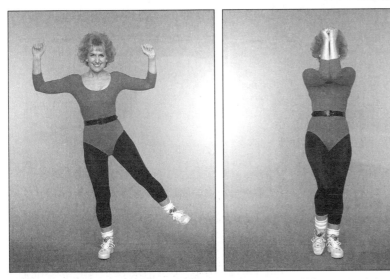

Raise alternate legs to the side with toes facing forwards and hips square, bringing your bent arms in and out at shoulder level. Do 32.

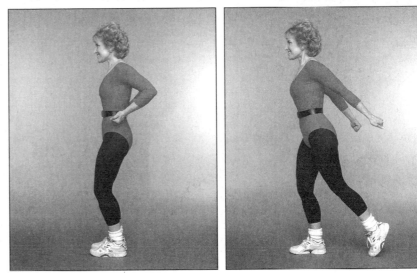

Keeping your elbows as far back and as close together as possible, tap alternate feet behind you, extending your arms to the back. Do 32.

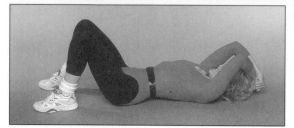

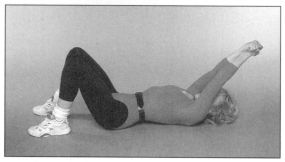

Upper Arm Toner Lying on the floor with knees bent, bend your arms and place them over your head. Straighten the arms, then bend them again. Repeat this movement 16–18 times.

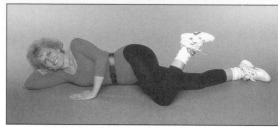

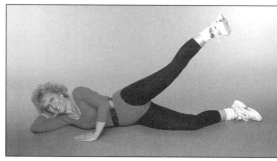

Outer Thigh Toner Lie on your side with both knees slightly bent. Dip the knee of the top leg on the floor in front and then, leading with the heel, extend and straighten it towards the corner of the room. Repeat this dipping and straightening movement 16–18 times, ensuring the hips remain square. Roll over, and repeat with the other leg.

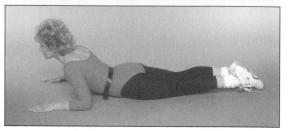

Back Strengthener Place your arms to the sides with elbows bent, palms facing upwards. Slowly raise your chest off the floor, using the muscles in your back not your arms. Return to the floor and repeat. Do 16–18.

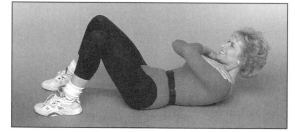

Tummy Toner Lie on your back with your knees bent and your hands placed across your chest. *Pulling your tummy in tightly*, raise your head and shoulders off the floor for a count of 2, then lower to a count of 2. Do 16–18.

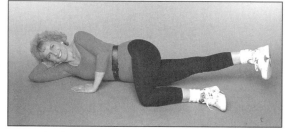

Inner Thigh Toner Lying on your side, bend the top leg and rest it on the floor in front of you. Keeping the bottom leg straight, lift it up and down 16–18 times. Roll over, and repeat with the other leg.

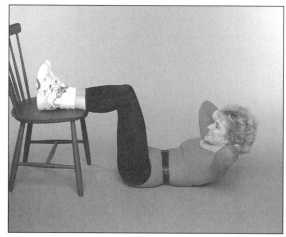

Tummy Toner Lie on your back with your feet placed against a wall or on a sturdy chair, and support your head with your hands. *Pulling your tummy in tightly*, raise your head and shoulders off the floor, keeping a distance between your chin and your chest. Raise on a count of 2, and return to the floor on a count of 2. Repeat 16–18 times.

Inner Thigh Stretch Sit up with knees bent and soles of the feet together. Using your elbows, gently ease your knees down as far as is comfortable. Hold for 15 seconds.

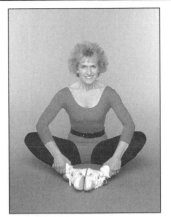

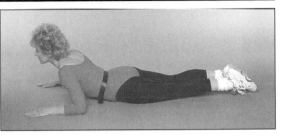

Tummy Stretch Lying face down, place your arms to the sides with elbows bent. Slowly raise your head and shoulders off the floor, supporting yourself on your forearms and elbows, and feel the stretch down the front of your abdomen. Hold for 10 seconds.

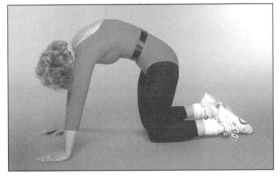

Back Stretch Position yourself on all fours and arch the spine as much as possible, pulling your tummy towards your spine. Hold for 10 seconds.

Back of Upper Arm Stretch Raise one elbow and ease your hand down your back. Use the other arm to ease it further. Hold for 10 seconds. Repeat with the other arm.

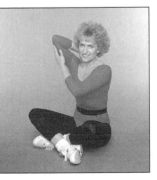

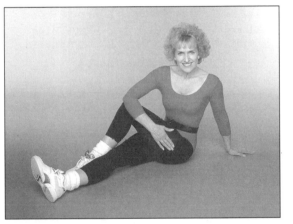

Outer Thigh Stretch Sit with one leg extended and the other leg placed across it with foot flat on the floor approximately level with the knee of the straight leg. Use the opposite elbow to ease the bent knee across, and hold for 10 seconds. Relax, then change position to repeat with the other leg.

POSITIVE THOUGHT FOR THE DAY

For exercise to become a habit, we need to find ways of exercising that we enjoy. Having reached this stage of the plan and having undertaken the daily exercise routines, you will no doubt realise how much better you feel and how much more energy you have. Exercise is such a positive activity and can greatly help to improve our general health and well-being. Some people who have physically demanding jobs may think that they do not need any additional exercise. This is not necessarily so. They may be undertaking 'workercise', which is repetitive, using just a few muscles and joints most of the time doing the physical tasks their job demands. However, what our body needs is a good all-round balanced workout. 'Funercise' activities like swimming and jogging, playing ball or walking benefit the whole body and are also sociable. Often we have bad memories of exercise from our school days. If you were made to run across country and hated every minute of it you probably feel less inclined to go on a jog in the countryside now. You have these deeply engraved bad memories that are negative, full of anger, discomfort and humiliation. Try to overcome these by putting yourself into a physically active environment you enjoy. Acknowledge the fact that there is *no* pressure and that you are doing it because you *want* to. Start seeing the great *benefits* and not the discomforts of such an activity. Start undertaking a new activity today and do it in *addition* to the set workout each day to the end of the 28-day plan. If you wish, do a different activity *every* day. On the days it's not convenient for you to go out, just walk up and down the stairs 20 or 30 times, and realise what a great workout you can have without even leaving your home or office!

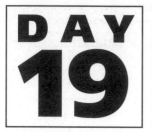

We must be realistic about the body we have. There is no point in our craving a waif-like body similar to the models we see in *Vogue*. Such models are usually underweight. The average person is not going to get that thin, and most of us would look ghastly if we did. We can, however, make the very best of ourselves and achieve slimness not thinness and become fit without becoming fanatical. Taking the steps you have made so far on this diet and fitness plan has given you the best possible start in learning how to build confidence, how to eat healthily and exercise safely and how to maintain this new lifestyle in the long term.

How long ago did you restyle your hair? As we gain confidence in our appearance we can be bolder in the style of clothes we choose and wear more confident colours. Start working towards the new wardrobe you will be wanting to build after you have reached the end of the 28 days or beyond, depending on how much weight you have to lose. Planning a new wardrobe is very exciting and won't happen instantly. Consider having a colour analysis to find what colours suit you best. It is quite staggering to realise how certain colours make us look vibrant and healthy while others make us look as though we died yesterday! Look in the telephone book for details of your nearest consultant.

Enjoy today's exercises and the exciting new recipes that have been included today. Only two more days before your next weighing and measuring session, so stick with it and no cheating! Enjoy yourself.

MENU

BREAKFAST

3 fl oz (75 ml) orange juice; 3 x 5 oz (125 g) diet yogurts, any flavour, plus 1 piece fresh fruit

or

8 oz (200 g) smoked haddock, microwaved or steamed, served with 1 slice light bread

LUNCH

℗ 2 slices wholemeal bread, filled with 2 oz (50 g) tuna (in brine) and 2 oz (50 g) low-fat cottage cheese, plus sliced tomato

Ⓠ 1 x 16 oz (400 g) can Heinz Farmhouse Potato and Leek Soup, with 1 slice wholemeal toast (no butter) plus 1 x 5 oz (125 g) diet yogurt

Toasted Sandwich

Ⓡ 2 slices wholemeal bread toasted and filled with 2 oz (50 g) turkey rashers and dry-fried onions. Serve with side salad of chopped lettuce, spinach, endive, tomato, red and green pepper 4 oz (100 g) fresh fruit

DINNER

STARTER
Tomato and Orange Soup
(page 159)

Ⓡ *Lamb Kebabs with Onion Sauce*
(page 161)

Ⓠ 5 oz (125 g) pork steak (all fat removed) grilled and served with unlimited vegetables plus 2 oz (50 g) apple sauce made without sugar

Ⓥ *Vegetarian Loaf* (page 174)

DESSERT
Pears in Meringue (page 177)

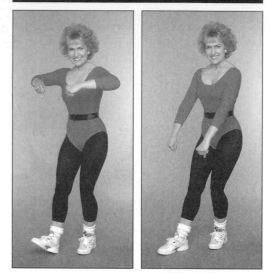

Tap the toes of one foot to the floor 8 times while punching down with your arms. Repeat with the other foot.

Roll both shoulders backwards while transferring your weight from one foot to the other. Do 16.

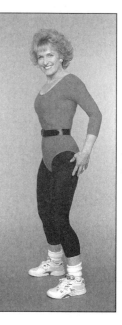

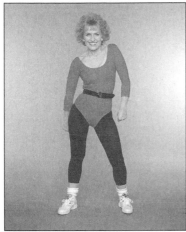

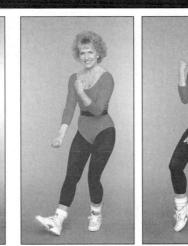

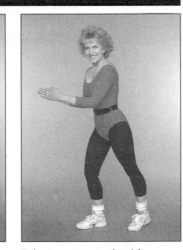

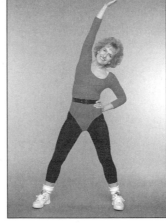

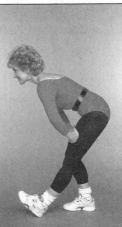

Back of Thigh Stretch Bend one knee and, keeping your weight on that foot, extend the other leg in front, toes raised. Feel the stretch at the back of the knee and the thigh. Hold for 10 seconds, then change legs and repeat.

With feet a comfortable distance apart, raise one hip and at the same time raise the opposite shoulder. Repeat with the other hip and shoulder. Do 16 on alternate sides.

Tap the heel and then the toe of one foot, flexing and straightening alternate arms. Do 8, then repeat with the other foot.

Take two steps to the side, moving your arms in a 'train-like' motion as you step. Repeat to the other side. Do 16 to alternate sides.

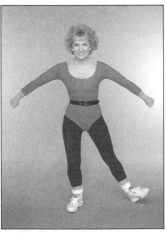

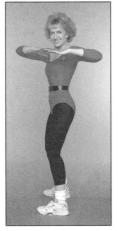

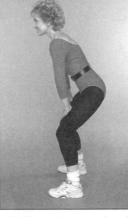

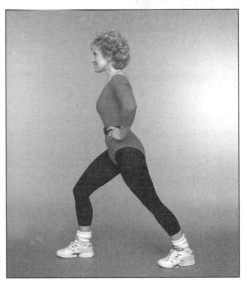

Extend alternate legs to the side, tapping the floor with your heels and swinging your arms in and out. Do 16.

Keeping the hips square, twist your upper body from side to side. Do not jerk. Do 8 to each side.

With feet wide apart, bend your knees and go down into a squat, ensuring knees bend over ankles. Come up again, and repeat. Do 8.

With one arm raised, lean directly to the side. Return to the starting position, and repeat to the other side. Do 8 to each side.

Calf Stretch Shift your weight on to the front leg and bend the knee. Your back leg is straight, heel on the floor and toes of both feet facing straight ahead. Keep your weight slightly forwards and feel the stretch in the calf muscle of your back leg. Hold for 10 seconds, then change legs and repeat.

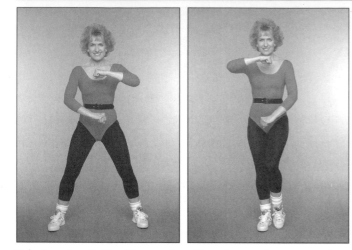 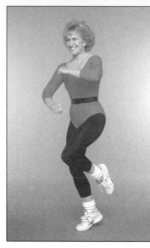 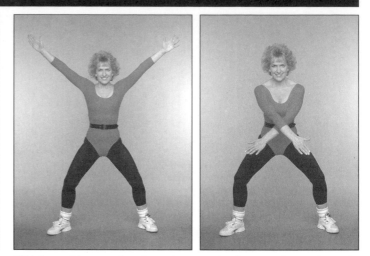

Take two steps to the side, pressing alternate arms down as you step. Repeat to the other side. Do 16 to alternate sides.

Jog on the spot and beat an imaginary drum. Keep your knees soft and bring your heels down as you land. Do 32.

With feet wide apart, bend your knees and make sweeping circles with your arms. Do 24.

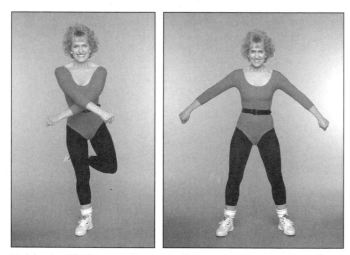 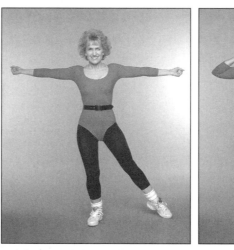 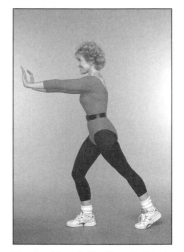

Kick back with alternate feet, swinging your arms out and in and crossing them in front. Do 32.

Touch alternate feet to the side, pointing your toes and bending and straightening your arms at shoulder level. Do 32.

Step and touch the floor behind with alternate feet, pushing your hands forwards as you take each foot back. Do 32.

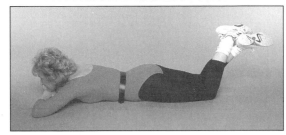

Back of Thigh Toner Lie face down and cross your ankles. Bend your knees and slowly raise your ankles, using the resistance of the top leg to make the exercise more difficult. Lower, and repeat. Do 14–16. Repeat with the other ankle on top.

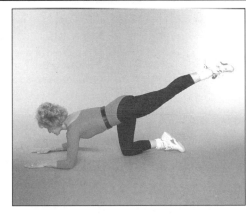

Bottom Toner Resting your weight on your forearms, extend one leg behind you. Keeping the leg straight, raise it in line with your hips – no higher – then lower it again. Raise and lower the leg 14–16 times, keeping your tummy in and your back flat throughout. Repeat with the other leg.

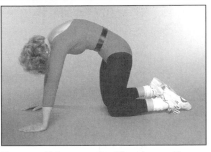

Tummy Trimmer Position yourself on all fours and pull your tummy muscles in as tightly as you can to arch your spine. Relax, and repeat 14–16 times.

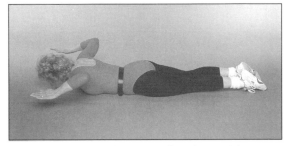

Upper Back Strengthener Lie face down with arms bent at shoulder level. Raise your arms, squeezing your shoulder blades together as much as possible. Lower your arms, and repeat. Do 14–16.

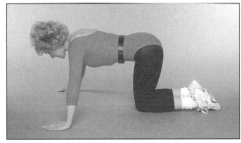

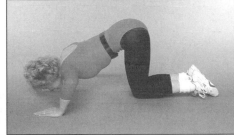

Chest Toner Position yourself on all fours with your hands placed on the floor slightly wider than shoulder-width apart. Slowly lower your head to the floor, then lift up again, keeping your chin in line with your hands. Keep your tummy tight and your back straight throughout. Repeat 14–16 times.

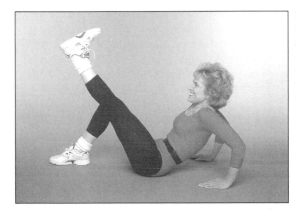

Front Thigh Toner Sit up with both legs bent, and support your weight on your hands. Straighten one leg and raise it to the level of the other knee, then lower it again. Do 14–16 straight leg lifts, keeping your tummy tight. Repeat with the other leg.

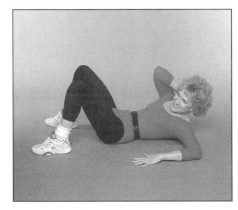

Waist Toner Lying on your back with both knees bent, place one hand behind your neck and have the other arm on the floor for support. Raise your head and shoulder and bring your elbow towards the opposite knee, taking care not to roll your hips. Return to the floor, and repeat. Do 16–18, then repeat to the other side.

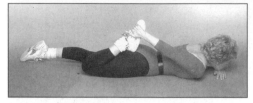

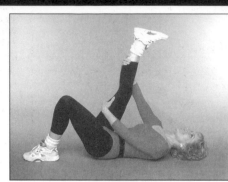

Front Thigh Stretch Lie on your front and rest your head on one hand. Bend the opposite leg and use your hand to ease it towards your seat. Hold for 10 seconds then release, and repeat with the other leg.

Back of Thigh Stretch Lie on your back with knees bent. Take hold of one leg and raise it, straightening it as far as is comfortable. Ease the leg towards you with your hands and hold for 10–15 seconds. Relax, and repeat with the other leg.

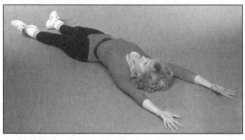

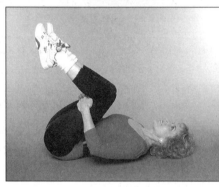

Full Body Stretch Lie on your back and extend your arms and legs as much as possible. Hold for 10 seconds.

Seat Stretch Bend your knees towards your chest and place your hands underneath your thighs. Ease your legs further towards your chest and feel the stretch in your seat. Hold for 10 seconds.

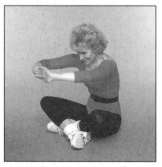

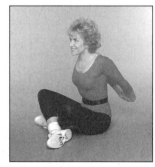

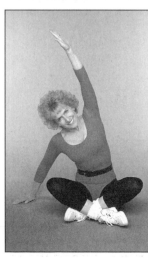

Upper Back Stretch Sitting with legs crossed, round your back and raise your arms in front to shoulder level to separate your shoulder blades. Hold for 10 seconds.

Chest Stretch Raise your arms and clasp your hands behind your back to stretch the muscles across your chest. Hold for 10 seconds.

Waist Stretch Place one hand on the floor for support, and reach over to the side with the other arm. Hold for 10 seconds, then relax and repeat to the other side.

POSITIVE THOUGHT FOR THE DAY

Many people think that they don't have time to exercise, but the truth is that we just can't afford not to make the time. By eliminating the harmful effects of mental stress, a well-designed exercise programme undertaken regularly will improve the quality of your sleep and increase your alertness. It will vastly improve your attitude and it will help put any difficulties that you may have into perspective. It's interesting to note that people who undertake regular exercise rarely suffer from depression. No matter what your job is, you will find that if you exercise regularly the quality of your decisions will improve and your productivity will increase. Set yourself goals, but keep them realistic. Start gently and gradually build up. Getting into an exercise discipline is extremely rewarding mentally and the feeling of 'I actually did it' is so tremendous that it really does set you up for the rest of the day. When I first started to take our two dogs for an early morning run each day it was tough to maintain the discipline during the first few weeks, but it soon became an enjoyable routine. The effect on my body was most encouraging and that really spurred me on to continue. Getting fit and toned doesn't happen overnight but it's worth working at. Once you accomplish it, you can hang on to that fitter, firmer body without doing too much to maintain it. It's just taking that original decision to make the effort. When you do, you'll be glad you did.

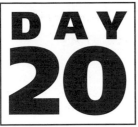

DAY 20

Try on your skirt or pair of trousers and see how much looser it is. It's been several days since you tried it on and you should see a significant difference. It always seems extraordinary to fathom what actually happens to the fat. But the best way that I can describe it is to think of a log burning on a fire. It produces heat and disappears to almost nothing, just a few ashes. Similarly, the fat we burn off our body produces heat and disappears into thin air. By following a low-fat diet and taking regular exercise you will find that you lose weight at a sensible rate so that the skin shrinks as you shed your inches, preventing flabby skin. Exercise will definitely help to encourage your skin to shrink and to give you a beautifully formed body at the end of your weight-loss campaign, leaving no signs that you were ever overweight in the first place. Nicole Blount, who lost eight stone (58.1 kg) and featured in my *New You Plan* and *Flat Stomach Plan* videos, exercised every day during the eight months that she dieted. By so doing, she was able to burn fat and tone up her body simultaneously. A combination of my Hip and Thigh diet and her daily workout to the video gave her the passport to a perfect body. No one would ever guess that she had been 16 stone (116.1 kg).

Now, what about you? People must be noticing your progress. Learn to accept their compliments and enjoy your success. Be extra good today and try to be as physically active as possible. Enjoy the exercises and try not to falter on the diet.

MENU

BREAKFAST

¼ pint/5 fl oz (125 ml) orange juice; 2 slices (3 oz/75 g) wholemeal bread spread with Marmite

or

As much fresh fruit as you can eat at one sitting

LUNCH

℗ Tuna and Pasta Salad

Mix 4 oz (100 g) [cooked weight] pasta twirls with 2 oz (50 g) tuna (in brine), 2 tbsp reduced-oil salad dressing and 2 oz (50 g) sweetcorn. Serve with a green salad
1 x 5 oz (125 g) diet yogurt

Q 3 oz (75 g) sardines in tomato sauce drained and served on 1 slice wholemeal toast. Serve with green salad (lettuce, peppers, endive) sprinkled with lemon juice

R 8 oz (200 g) jacket potato topped with 2 oz (50 g) low-fat cottage cheese mixed with chopped green and red peppers and 3 oz (75 g) sweetcorn

DINNER

STARTER
Creamy Vegetable Soup
(page 158)

R 6 oz (150 g) roast chicken, served with Dry-roast Potatoes (page 175), sage and onion stuffing and unlimited vegetables and gravy

Q Pork Casserole (page 167)

V Vegetable Kebabs (page 174)

DESSERT
2 pieces any fresh fruit

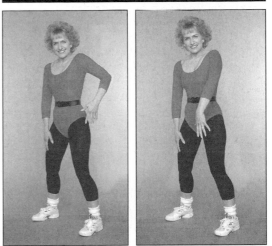

Roll alternate shoulders backwards, transferring your weight from one foot to the other. Do 16, then repeat, rolling shoulders forwards.

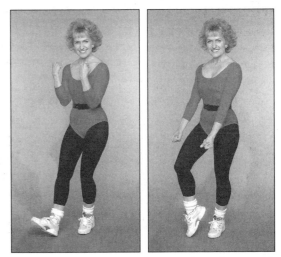

Tap the heel and then the toe of one foot, flexing and straightening both arms. Do 8, then repeat with the other foot.

CONTINUED ▶

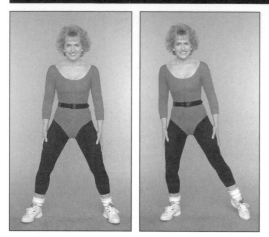

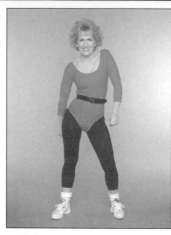

With feet a comfortable distance apart, transfer your weight from one foot to the other, bending your knees and tapping the toes of the opposite foot as you step. Do 16.

With feet a comfortable distance apart, raise one hip and at the same time raise the opposite shoulder. Repeat with the other hip and shoulder. Do 16 on alternate sides.

Transferring your weight from one foot to the other, swing alternate arms in complete circles. Do 16.

Back of Thigh Stretch Bend one knee and, keeping your weight on that foot, extend the other leg in front, toes raised. Feel the stretch at the back of the knee and the thigh. Hold for 10 seconds, then change legs and repeat.

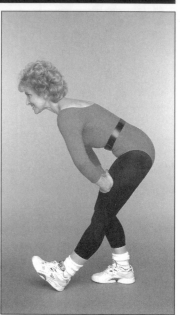

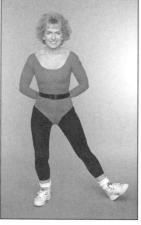

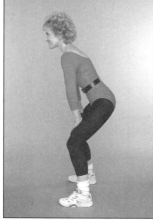

With one arm raised, palm facing upwards, and the other hand on your hip, lean directly to the side, reaching over with the raised arm. Do not twist the hips. Return to the starting position and repeat to the other side. Do 8 to each side.

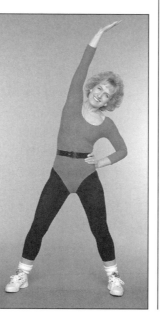

Extend alternate legs to the side, tapping the floor with your heels. Do 16.

With feet wide apart, bend your knees and go down into a squat, making sure the knees bend over the ankles. Come up again, and repeat. Do 8.

Calf Stretch Shift your weight on to the front leg and bend the knee. Your back leg is straight, heel on the floor and toes of both feet facing straight ahead. Keep your weight slightly forwards and feel the stretch in the calf muscle of your back leg. Hold for 10 seconds, then change legs and repeat.

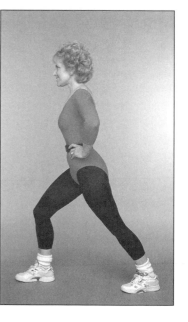

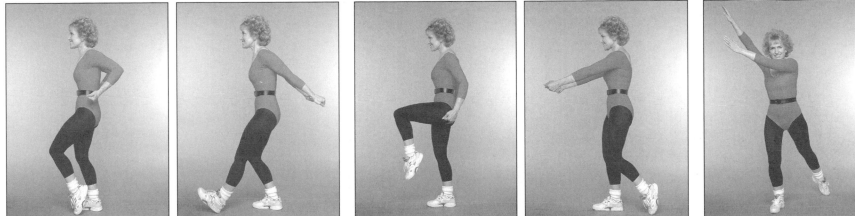

With elbows bent and raised behind you, tap the toes and then the heel of one foot, straightening your arms behind you as you tap. Keep your elbows as high as possible. Repeat with the other foot. Do 32 with alternate feet.

Raise one knee in front, then tap the toes behind, bringing the arms backwards and forwards as if pulling drawers out and in. Keep your tummy tight throughout. Do 32, then repeat with the other leg.

Step with one foot and touch the other foot to the floor behind on a diagonal, swinging your arms high to the side. Repeat to the other side. Do 24.

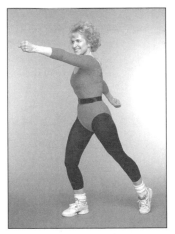

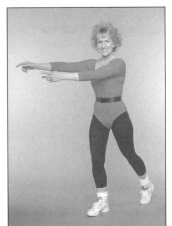

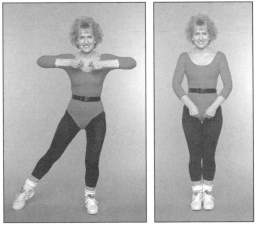

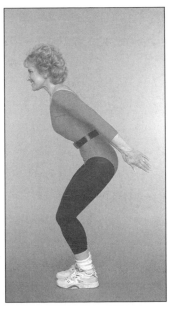

Step and touch behind with alternate feet, swinging alternate arms forwards and backwards. Do 24.

Extend alternate legs on a diagonal to touch the floor behind, swinging your arms from side to side. Do 32.

Extend alternate legs to the side, pointing your toes and bending and straightening your arms up and down in front. Do 32.

Stand with knees together, feet facing straight ahead and arms stretched above your head. Ski down, bending your knees and swinging your arms down and to the back of you. Return to the starting position, and repeat, keeping your chest lifted throughout. Do 32.

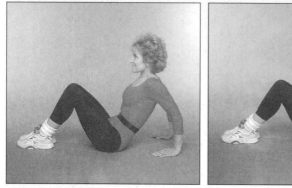

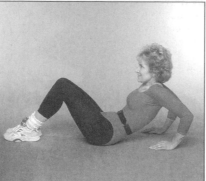

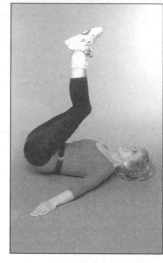

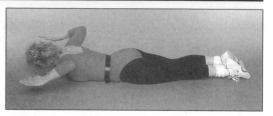

Upper Arm Toner Sit with knees bent and prop yourself up on your hands. Your hands should be placed at least 12 inches (30 cm) behind your back, with fingers pointing forwards. Bend your arms so that your elbows move backwards, then straighten them again. Do 16–18.

Upper Back Strengthener Lie face down with arms bent at shoulder level. Raise your arms, squeezing your shoulder blades together as much as possible, then lower your arms. Repeat 16–18 times.

Tummy Trimmer Lie on your back with legs raised and slightly bent. Your feet are over your hips and your tummy is pulled in tightly. Press your tummy muscles down and lift the hips slightly off the floor. Repeat 16–18 times, ensuring the effort comes from your abdomen, not your arms.

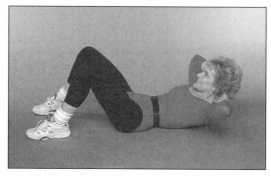

Tummy Toner Lie on your back with knees bent and your *tummy pulled in tightly*. Place your hands behind your neck and slowly raise your head and shoulders off the floor. Raise on a count of 2, then return to the floor on a count of 2. Do 16–18.

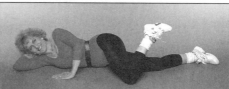

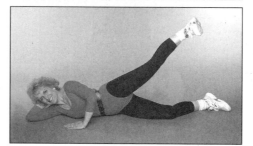

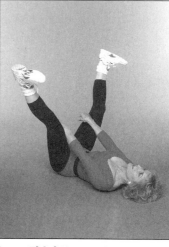

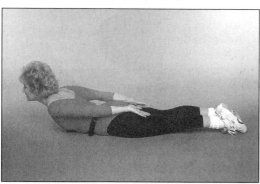

Back Strengthener Lie face down with your hands placed on your seat. Slowly raise your chest and shoulders off the floor, using the muscles in your spine. Return to the floor, and repeat. Do 8–10.

Outer Thigh Toner Lie on your side with both knees slightly bent. Dip the knee of the top leg on the floor in front and then, leading with the heel, extend and straighten it towards the corner of the room. Repeat this dipping and straightening movement 16–18 times, ensuring the hips remain square. Roll over, and repeat with the other leg.

Inner Thigh Toner Lie on your back with your feet raised above your hips, legs apart, and hands on the inside of your thighs. Use your hands for resistance as you aim to bring your legs together. Keep your back pressed into the floor. Do 16–18.

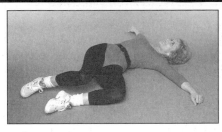

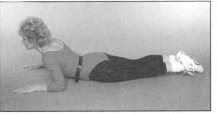

Outer Thigh Stretch Lying your back with arms outstretched and knees bent, lower both knees slowly to one side, keeping both feet on the floor. Hold for 10 seconds. Slowly raise the knees to the centre, and repeat to the other side.

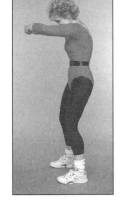

Tummy Stretch Lie face down with arms bent. Slowly raise your head and shoulders off the floor, supporting yourself on your forearms and elbows, and feel the stretch down the front of your abdomen. Hold for 10 seconds.

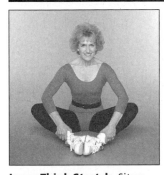

Inner Thigh Stretch Sit up with knees bent and soles of the feet together. Using your elbows, gently ease your knees down as far as is comfortable. Hold for 15 seconds.

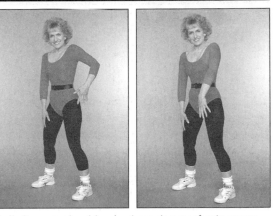

Roll alternate shoulders backwards, transferring your weight from one foot to the other. Do 16, then repeat, this time rolling shoulders forwards.

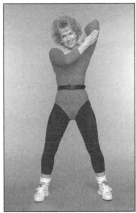

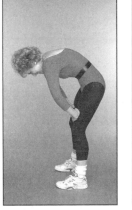

Back of Upper Arm Stretch Standing with feet a comfortable distance apart and knees slightly bent, raise one elbow and ease your hand down your back, using the other arm to assist. Hold for 10 seconds. Relax, and repeat with the other arm.

Back Stretch Rest your hands on your thighs, just above your knees, to support your weight. Arch your back as much as possible, pulling your tummy in, and feel the stretch down your back. Hold for 10 seconds.

Upper Back Stretch Round your back and raise your arms in front to shoulder level to separate your shoulder blades. Hold for 10 seconds.

POSITIVE THOUGHT FOR THE DAY

A few days ago we were looking at not putting people down. It's equally important not to put ourselves down. There are lots of people out there who will do it for us so there's no need for us to do it as well. We often knock ourselves on the basis that if we say something negative about ourselves first, then nobody else will say it to us, and if *we* say it somebody might even argue and say that it isn't true. Many of us are not very good at acknowledging our strengths. For instance, so often we are unable to accept a compliment in the spirit in which it is intended. A friend says to you after dining at your home, 'That was the most delicious meal I have ever tasted,' yet how many of us say, 'Oh well, it was nothing. It was just out of a packet.' Instead we should say, 'Thank you, I'm glad you enjoyed it.' If we wear a new dress or suit and somebody comments favourably on our appearance we tend to reply 'I only bought it in the sale' or some other ungracious comment. Why do we do it? We should learn to accept a compliment and say, 'Thank you, that's very kind.' It makes the deliverer of the compliment feel happier and it shows great confidence from us.

I know we shouldn't take ourselves too seriously but there is a world of difference between laughing at ourselves over some small situation and knocking our abilities, courage, common sense, enthusiasm and steadiness. You must learn to believe in yourself. Start learning to like yourself and come to terms with the minor imperfections that you may see. If you have insufficient self respect or belief in yourself, how on earth can you expect other people to respect you either? Start showing signs of confidence and try to take on board the fact that you are the best person you know!

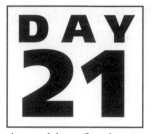

DAY 21

When you started the diet three weeks ago did you honestly believe that you would find enough willpower to be able to stay the course and to be able to see the real benefits that I said you would enjoy? By making this effort you will be able to look forward to the rest of your life with new confidence and a new feeling of belief and determination for the future. You have shown enormous dedication so far and tomorrow is weighing and measuring day. Today, aim to be as physically active as possible and really aim to maximise your weight and inch loss by tomorrow. Try to undertake some additional physical activity – going swimming with the family or taking the dog for a long, brisk walk. Do two activities if you have time! Perform the exercises carefully and realise just how much progress you have made since you started them three weeks ago. You should be feeling stronger, fitter, more flexible and have much greater stamina. Well done. Be a paragon of virtue today and look forward to the scales and tape measure being kind to you tomorrow.

MENU

BREAKFAST

4 fl oz (100 ml) orange juice; 1/2 ogen melon, deseeded and chopped, served with 5 oz (125 g) diet yogurt, any flavour
or
3 green figs plus 5 oz (125 g) diet yogurt

LUNCH

P 4 slices light bread spread with Marmite and filled with 4 oz (100 g) low-fat cottage cheese; 1 piece fresh fruit

Q 4 brown Ryvitas topped with 4 oz (100 g) tuna (in brine) mixed with 1 tbsp reduced-oil salad dressing, plus mixed salad

R *Fresh Fruit Medley*
4 oz (100 g) strawberries, 4 oz (100 g) raspberries, 4 oz (100 g) cherries, 4 oz (100 g) redcurrants or blackcurrants mixed with 1 tsp honey and 8 oz (200 g) Müllerlight raspberry or strawberry flavour yogurt

DINNER

STARTER
Corn on the cob (frozen or tinned)

R *Cod in Parsley Sauce* (page 168)

Q 1/2 can (8 oz/200 g) Princes Stewed Steak with Gravy, served with unlimited vegetables

V *Spiced Bean Casserole* (page 171)

DESSERT
4 fl oz (100 ml) orange juice; 2 oz (50 g) Wall's 'Too Good To Be True' ice cream sprinkled with 1/2 oz (12.5 g) Bran Flakes or Fruit 'n Fibre

Rotate your hips in a clockwise direction. Do 8, then repeat in an anti-clockwise direction.

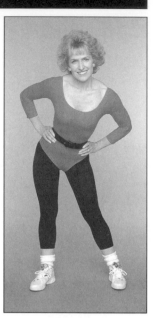

Roll both shoulders forwards, transferring your weight from one foot to the other. Do 16.

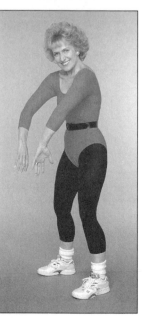

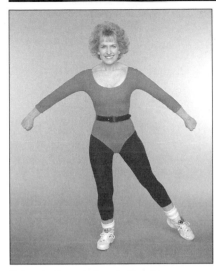

Extend alternate legs to the side, pointing your toes and swinging your arms in and out as you step. Do 16.

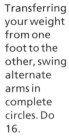

Transferring your weight from one foot to the other, swing alternate arms in complete circles. Do 16.

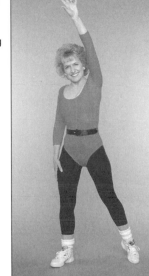

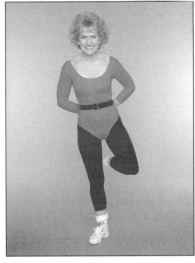

Kick back with alternate feet. Do 16.

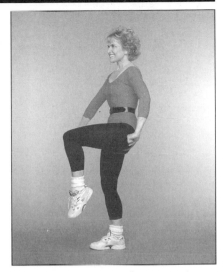

Raise alternate knees in front, pressing down with both arms. Keep your tummy tight and back straight. Do 16.

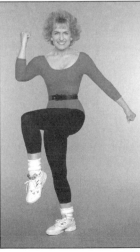

Raise alternate knees and aim to touch with opposite elbow. Do 16.

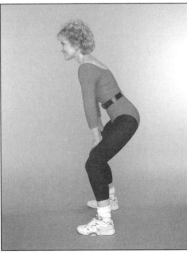

With feet wide apart, bend your knees and go down into a squat, making sure the knees bend over the ankles. Come up again, and repeat. Do 8.

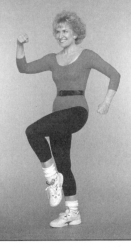

March on the spot, swinging your arms strongly. Don't stamp. Do 32.

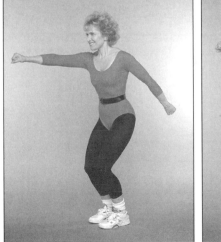

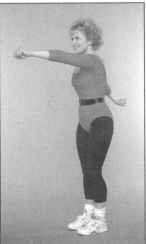

With feet together, dip down, bending your knees and then straightening them, swinging alternate arms forwards and backwards. Do 32.

CONTINUED ▶

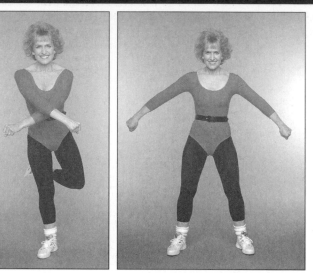

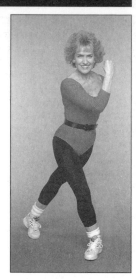

Step and curtsey, taking alternate feet behind and pressing opposite arms across your chest as your step. Do 32.

Kick back with alternate feet, swinging your arms out and in and crossing them in front. Do 32.

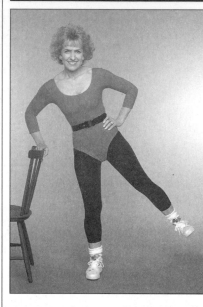

Outer Thigh Toner Stand and hold on to the back of a chair. Raise the outside leg out to the side, keeping your hips square and toes pointing forwards. Lower the leg, and repeat. Do 16–18, then turn round and repeat with the other leg.

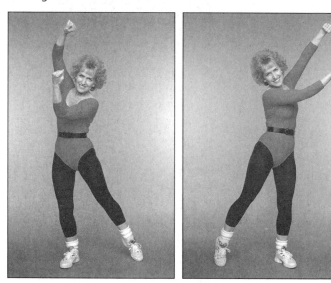

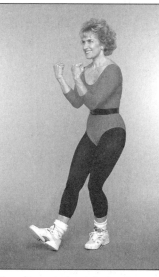

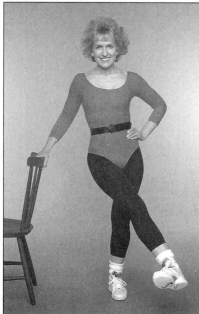

Inner Thigh Toner Extend the inside leg forwards and across the body then back again. Keep your hips square. Do 16–18, then turn round and repeat with the other leg.

Step and touch alternate feet to the side, swinging your arms in a figure of eight as you step. Do 32.

Tap alternate heels in front, flexing and straightening both arms as you step. Do 32.

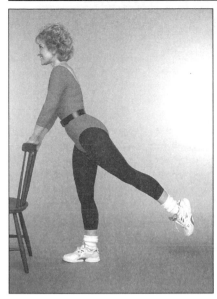

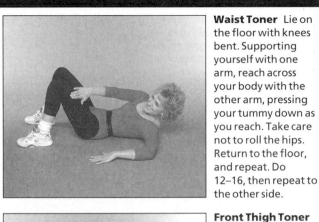

Waist Toner Lie on the floor with knees bent. Supporting yourself with one arm, reach across your body with the other arm, pressing your tummy down as you reach. Take care not to roll the hips. Return to the floor, and repeat. Do 12–16, then repeat to the other side.

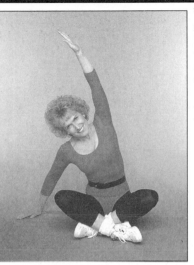

Waist Stretch Sit with legs crossed, and place one hand on the floor for support. Reach over to the side with the other arm. Hold for 10 seconds, then relax and repeat to the other side.

Bottom Toner Face the chair and raise one leg behind you, keeping the leg straight and squeezing your seat as you raise. Lower the leg, and repeat. Keep your tummy tight, hips square and your back straight throughout. Do 16–18, then repeat with the other leg.

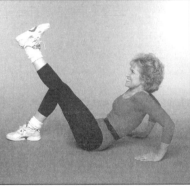

Front Thigh Toner Sit up with both legs bent, and support your weight on your hands. Straighten one leg and raise it to the level of the other knee, then lower it again. Do 16–18 straight leg lifts, keeping your tummy tight. Repeat with the other leg.

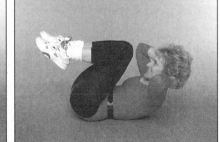

Tummy Streamliner Lie on your back with knees bent and raised over your hips, and place your hands on either side of your head. *Pull your tummy in tightly* and lift your head and shoulders and, at the same time, bring your knees in towards your chest. Keep a distance between your chin and your chest. Return to the floor, and repeat. Do 16–18.

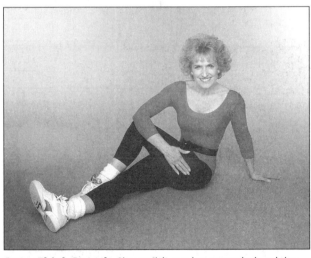

Outer Thigh Stretch Sit up with one leg extended and the other leg bent and placed across the straight leg approximately level with the knee. Use the opposite elbow to ease the bent knee across. Hold for 10 seconds. Relax, and change position and repeat with the other leg.

CONTINUED ▶

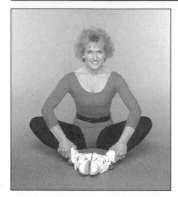

Inner Thigh Stretch Sit up with knees bent and soles of the feet together. Using your elbows, gently ease your knees down as far as is comfortable. Hold for 15 seconds.

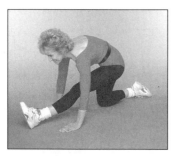

Back of Thigh Stretch Resting on one knee, extend the other leg forwards and take your weight on to your hands placed at either side of your front leg. Ease your seat back towards your heel, but don't sit on it. Feel the stretch at the back of the front leg, and hold for 10 seconds. Relax, then change legs, and repeat.

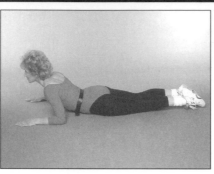

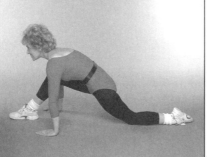

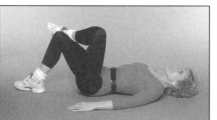

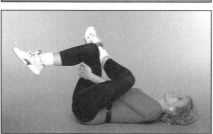

Tummy Stretch Lie face down with arms bent. Slowly raise your head and shoulders off the floor, supporting yourself on your forearms and elbows, and feel the stretch down the front of your abdomen. Hold for 10 seconds.

Upper Thigh Stretch Kneeling as shown, take your weight on to your front foot. Ease your hips forwards and feel the stretch in the front thigh of the back leg. Hold for 10 seconds, then relax, and repeat with the other leg.

Outer Thigh Stretch Lie on your back with knees bent. Cross one leg in front of the other knee. Place one hand through the middle of your legs and the other hand round the outside of the bottom leg. Slowly ease your legs towards your chest, and feel the stretch in the outer thigh of the top leg. Hold for 10 seconds, then relax and change legs to repeat on the other side.

POSITIVE THOUGHT FOR THE DAY

The end of your third week. Excellent! Success breeds confidence, so continue to build it up as each day goes by.

Everyone wants to believe in, depend on, be friends with and trust people who have confidence in themselves. A confident leader transmits confidence to her followers, and they *all* go forward. As soon as people lose confidence in their leader, everybody begins to doubt their *own* ability. If you want to be successful in *your* life the first barrier you have to demolish is your own lack of self-confidence. We build self-confidence by making sure that we 'win' often enough. Are you continuing to set yourself goals and are you achieving them? The more goals you set, the more you achieve and the more your confidence will grow. Don't set yourself unrealistic goals, but acknowledge your achievements no matter how small. When you feel confident that you are in control and you are a regular winner, then start setting higher goals, gradually move upwards and grow further.

In my exercise classes I am very much aware that people attending for the first time are often shy and uncomfortable, not knowing quite what to expect when they join the class. Feelings of am I going to be the heaviest, am I going to be able to do the exercises, is there going to be anyone of my age in the class? are all common thoughts. I try to make all my new members feel special and make an extra effort to remember their names. As they leave the class and I am able to say, 'Look forward to seeing you next week, Jane,' that person experiences several feelings. First, she will know that I have actually noted her in my memory. Second, she feels that I care, which of course I do, and third, she knows that she is going to be welcome next week. I remember these ladies by the leotards they wear or the group of friends that they are with. If I met the same ladies in the supermarket I might be struggling to remember their names, but as I have a fairly good memory of faces, I seem to get by. Remembering people's names is a habit that can be developed. Don't tell yourself that you're no good at it. This is a negative impulse and is really just an excuse for laziness. It's worth making the effort, as it makes people feel special.

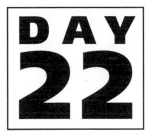

DAY 22

Three weeks under your belt and it's that big moment. Weigh and measure yourself and record your inch losses. Try on your skirt or trousers so you can really see the improvement you have made over the last three weeks. You must be feeling so pleased, not just because you have got this far with the programme but that you can actually see the results that you hoped for. Now you know it works and you have only one more week to go. Of course you can continue with the programme for as many weeks as you choose, selecting from the menus and performing whichever day's exercises you wish. But for now, we're looking at just one more week.

Now that you have a greater confidence in your body, start making plans to join a sports club perhaps, or take up a new hobby. The main reasons why people don't participate in sports activities is because they are shy, they don't regard themselves as sporty by nature, they feel overweight and they feel they lack energy. You don't feel any of these things now, so if you want to make exercise even more fun, seriously consider taking up a new activity.

During the last three weeks there have no doubt been times when you have been sorely tempted to cheat on the diet. *Remember* those feelings of temptation, and how you fought them. Are you glad that you did resist? It would be an awful shame if during this last week you were to put all that effort to waste. So please, gather up your willpower and march forward into this final furlong of the race. Enjoy today's activities and menus. Have a great day.

MENU

BREAKFAST

1 oz (25 g) Special K, 3 oz (75 g) chopped strawberries and 2 oz (50 g) grapes plus 3 fl oz (75 ml) milk (in addition to allowance)

or

1 whole fresh grapefruit; 1 rasher lean bacon grilled and made into a sandwich with 2 slices light bread spread with mustard or tomato ketchup

LUNCH

Ⓟ Tuna or Salmon Pitta

1 wholemeal pitta bread filled with 2 oz (50 g) tuna (in brine) or salmon and shredded lettuce, sliced tomato, cucumber, onion and pepper

Ⓠ 1 Golden Wonder 'Pot Light' Italian Chicken 1 piece fresh fruit

Ⓡ Jacket Potato with Onion Mushrooms
(page 160)

DINNER

STARTER
Chicken Liver Pâté with Brandy
(page 156)

Ⓡ Tasty Pork with Pasta (page 167)

Ⓠ Findus Lean Cuisine Kashmiri Chicken Curry with Rice

Ⓥ Curried Chickpeas (page 170)

DESSERT
Sultana Cake (page 178)

With feet hip-width apart and knees slightly bent, shrug alternate shoulders 16 times.

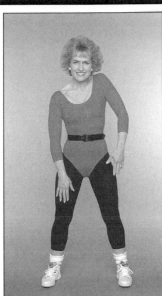

Rotate alternate arms backwards as if brushing your hair, transferring your weight from one foot to the other. Do 16.

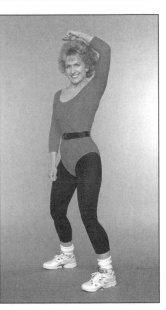

CONTINUED ▶

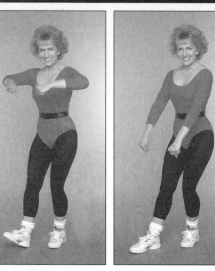
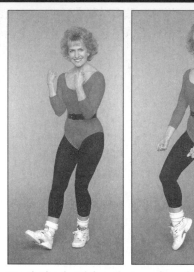
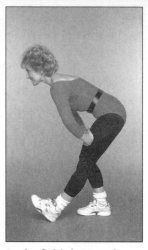

Tap the toes of one foot to the floor 8 times while punching down with your arms. Repeat with the other foot.

Tap the heel and then the toe of one foot, flexing and straightening both arms. Do 8, then repeat with the other foot.

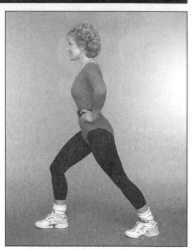

Back of Thigh Stretch
Bend one knee and, keeping your weight on that foot, extend the other leg in front, toes raised. Feel the stretch at the back of the knee and the thigh. Hold for 10 seconds, then change legs and repeat.

Calf Stretch Shift your weight on to the front leg and bend the knee. Your back leg is straight, heel on the floor and toes of both feet facing straight ahead. Keep your weight slightly forwards and feel the stretch in the calf muscle of your back leg. Hold for 10 seconds, then change legs and repeat.

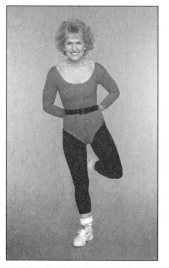
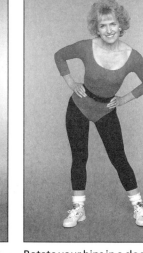

Kick back with alternate feet. Do 16.

Keeping the hips square, twist your upper body from side to side. Do not jerk. Do 8 to each side.

Rotate your hips in a clockwise direction. Do 8, then repeat in an anti-clockwise direction.

Front Thigh Stretch
Stand and hold on to the back of a chair. Keeping your inside leg slightly bent, bend the other leg and take hold of your foot. Ease the foot back and up, keeping both knees aligned. Hold for 10 seconds. Release, then turn round and repeat with the other leg.

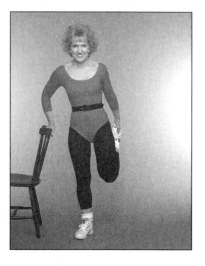

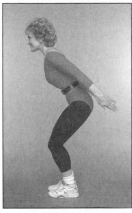 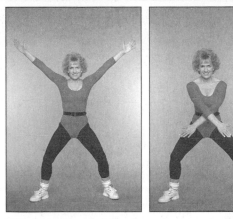 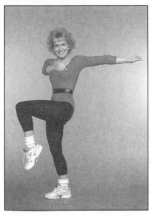 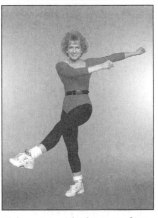 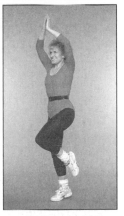

Stand with knees together, feet facing straight ahead and arms stretched above your head. Ski down, bending your knees and swinging your arms down. Come up again and repeat.

With feet wide apart, bend your knees and make sweeping circles with your arms. Do 24.

Keeping your tummy pulled in throughout, raise alternate knees across your body, swinging your arms from side to side. Do 24.

Kick across with alternate feet, swinging your arms from side to side in the opposite direction to your feet. Do 32.

Jog on the spot, lifting your legs high behind you and clapping your hands above your head. Keep your knees soft and bring your heels down as you land. Do 32.

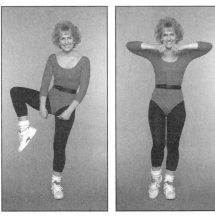 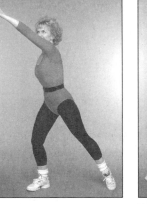 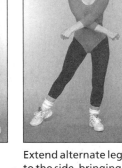 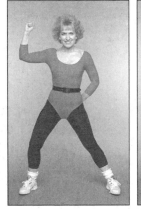 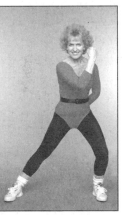

Raise alternate knees out to the side, pushing your arms down and up in 'barrow boy' style as you step. Do 24.

Step and lunge to one side, reaching across with opposite arm. Only the toes of the straight leg should touch the floor. Try to straighten the arm and leg as much as possible as you lunge. Repeat to the other side. Do 32 to alternate sides.

Extend alternate legs to the side, bringing your arms out and in to cross in front. Do 32.

With feet wide apart, lunge from side to side, pressing the opposite arm across your body. Exert as much pressure as possible with each arm as you move from side to side. Do 32.

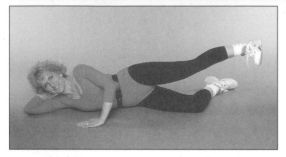

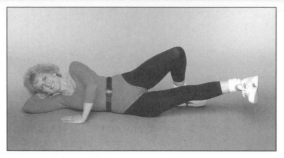

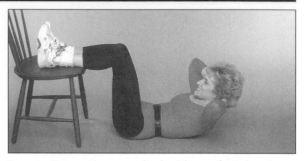

Outer Thigh Toner Lie on your side with your bottom leg bent and your top leg straight. Raise the top leg, keeping your hips square and your toes aiming slightly downwards. Do not raise the leg too high. Lower, then repeat. Do 16–18, then roll over and repeat with the other leg.

Inner Thigh Toner Bend the top leg and place the foot flat on the floor. Keeping the bottom leg straight, raise it as high as possible, making sure your hips remain square. Lower the leg, and repeat. Do 16–18, then roll over and repeat with the other leg.

Tummy Toner Lie on your back with your feet placed against a wall or on a sturdy chair, and support your head with your hands. *Pulling your tummy in tightly*, raise your head and shoulders off the floor, keeping a distance between your chin and your chest. Raise on a count of 2, and return to the floor on a count of 2. Repeat 16–18 times.

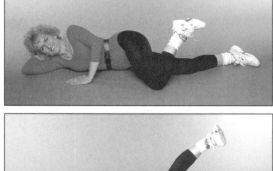

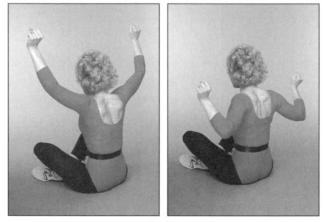

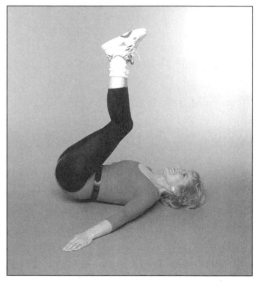

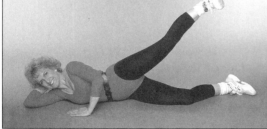

Upper Back Toner Sit upright with your legs crossed. Take your arms above your head and reach up. Now pull the elbows back and down to squeeze your shoulder blades together. Raise the arms again, and repeat. Do 16–18.

Outer Thigh Toner Lie on your side with both knees slightly bent. Dip the knee of the top leg on the floor in front and then, leading with the heel, extend and straighten it towards the corner of the room. Repeat this dipping and straightening movement 16–18 times, ensuring the hips remain square. Roll over, and repeat with the other leg.

Tummy Trimmer Lie on your back and raise your legs straight up towards the ceiling, ensuring your *feet are over your hips*. Press down with your tummy muscles and pull your legs towards your chest to lift your hips off the floor slightly. Don't use your arms to assist. Do 16–18.

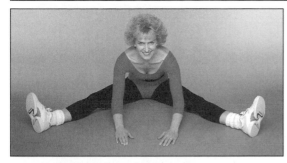

Advanced Inner Thigh Stretch Sitting with your legs wide apart and supporting your weight on your arms, ease your body forwards and feel the stretch in your inner thighs. Hold for 10 seconds.

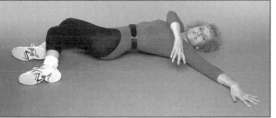

Waist and Outer Thigh Stretch Lying on your back with both knees bent, allow your knees to drop to one side while taking your arms to the opposite side. Hold for 10 seconds, then slowly return to the centre, and repeat to the other side.

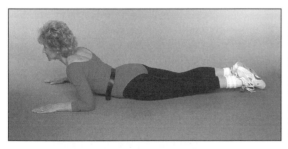

Tummy Stretch Lying face down with arms bent and legs together, slowly raise your head and shoulders off the floor, supporting yourself on your forearms and elbows. Feel the stretch down the front of your abdomen. Hold for 10 seconds.

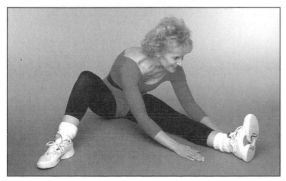

Back of Thigh Stretch Sitting with one leg straight and the other slightly bent, ease your weight forwards towards the straight leg and feel the stretch at the back of the knee and the thigh. Hold for 10 seconds, then change the position of the legs to repeat on the other side.

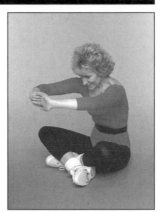

Upper Back Stretch Sitting with legs crossed, round your back and raise your arms in front to shoulder level to separate your shoulder blades. Hold for 10 seconds.

POSITIVE THOUGHT FOR THE DAY

In this last week of the 28-day plan I want to look at the one key ingredient to success. That key ingredient is self-discipline. Having self-discipline makes a huge difference to your everyday life. It affects your thinking, your planning, your hopes and your dreams because, unless you are able to discipline yourself in the direction that you want to grow, success will almost certainly elude you. Discipline is not something you're given or something you inherit. It is something that you acquire, and you will only acquire it if you realise how incredibly helpful it can be in improving your life.

Over the last few years as the demands on my time have become greater and greater, exercising self-discipline in my activities, in the food I eat, and in exercise has been vital. I believe self-discipline is the foundation of self-improvement. It channels our resources of time, energy and money into a habit of learning and growing towards something new and better each day. Another word for self-discipline is willpower. It's doing what you know you *should* do and avoiding what you know you should *not* do. Never is this so true as in the case of diet and exercise. We can *make* ourselves self-disciplined even if we haven't been that way in the past. It's never too late to make some changes. Start today by planning to make better use of your time each day. More about this tomorrow.

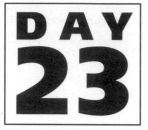

DAY 23

As you approach the end of this 28-day plan you will have learned a significant amount about low-fat eating by following the recipes that have been included so far. With this new-found knowledge, you'll find it easy to adapt your own favourite recipes by cutting out all additional fat and making a few substitutions. Remember, this programme is not a short-term solution, it is the beginning of a lifetime plan. Your fitter, stronger body is going to stand you in good stead for many years, giving you more energy than you ever imagined and enabling you to fulfil dreams that you thought were beyond you. I often receive letters from successful dieters telling me how their life has changed for the better. Some of the stories I read bring tears to my eyes, they are so heartwarming. There was the couple who wanted to adopt a baby and who were turned down on the grounds that the husband was six stone (43.5 kg) overweight. He lost his six stone on my diet in six months and, after four years of waiting patiently, they were given the most beautiful baby. If you have a story to tell me, please do not hesitate to write. I may include it in a future book and your story may inspire others to make the effort. That really is what *this* book is all about. Trying to encourage and inspire and keep the determination going.

The exercises today are even more challenging, but by now you should be so much stronger. Work hard on the toning exercises and feel the benefits. Enjoy today's menus and select something really tasty. You need to treat yourself in this last week as you go forward to the finishing line. Don't even think about cheating. Be saintly and be active.

MENU

BREAKFAST

3 fl oz (75 ml) orange juice; 1 x 8 oz (200 g) pot Müllerlight yogurt; 1 slice wholemeal toast spread with 2 tsp marmalade
or
6 oz (150 g) seedless grapes and 6 oz (150 g) chopped melon, topped with 5 oz (125 g) diet yogurt

LUNCH

Ⓟ Chicken Salad Sandwich
1 slice (1½ oz/37.5 g) wholemeal bread cut in half and filled with 2 oz (50 g) cooked chicken mixed with 2 tbsp Quark or low-fat fromage frais, plus shredded lettuce, sliced tomato and cucumber; 1 orange

Ⓞ 1 Heinz 'Lunchbowl' Lamb and Vegetable Casserole; 1 piece fresh fruit

Ⓡ Rice Salad
Cook 2 oz (50 g) [dry weight] brown rice and mix with 2 oz (50 g) cooked peas, 2 oz (50 g) canned red kidney beans, drained, 2 chopped spring onions and 2 tbsp oil-free French dressing. Top with 3 oz (75 g) low-fat cottage cheese

DINNER

STARTER
Watercress Soup (page 159)

Ⓡ Mediterranean Tuna Lasagne (page 168)

Ⓞ Chinese Menu 2 (page 162)
Singapore Beef Curry, Prawns in Yellow Bean Sauce, Chicken in Orange and Green Ginger Sauce

Ⓥ 1 vegeburger served with a sesame seed roll plus salad

DESSERT
6 oz (150 g) jelly with 2 oz (50 g) Wall's 'Too Good To Be True' ice cream

---

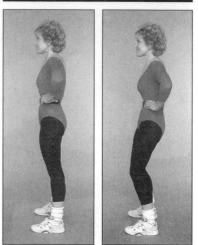

Stand in a good posture with your tummy in and your back straight, and tilt your pelvis forwards and upwards. Relax, and repeat. Do 8.

Roll both shoulders backwards while transferring your weight from one foot to the other. Do 16.

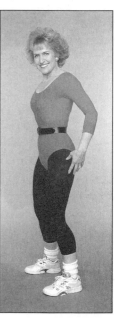

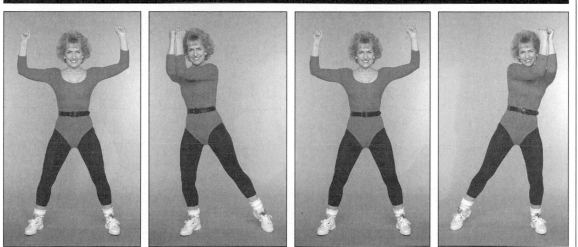

Step to alternate sides and touch opposite toes to the floor, bringing your bent arms in and out as you step. Do 32.

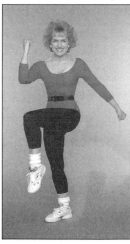
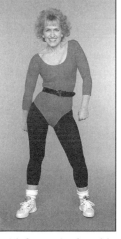
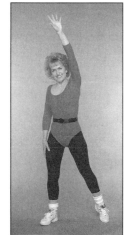
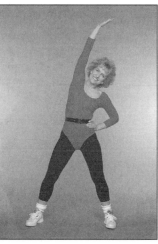

Raise alternate knees across and aim to touch with opposite elbow. Keep your tummy pulled in and your back straight. Do 32.

With feet a comfortable distance apart, raise one hip and at the same time raise the opposite shoulder. Repeat with the other hip and shoulder. Do 16 on alternate sides.

Transferring your weight from one foot to the other, swing alternate arms in complete circles. Do 16.

With feet a comfortable distance apart, lean directly to the side. Do not twist the hips. Return to the starting position, and repeat to the other side. Do 12 to each side.

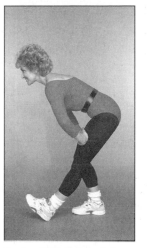
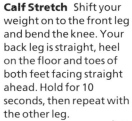

Back of Thigh Stretch Bend one knee and, keeping your weight on that foot, extend the other leg in front, toes raised. Feel the stretch at the back of the knee and the thigh. Hold for 10 seconds, then change legs and repeat.

Calf Stretch Shift your weight on to the front leg and bend the knee. Your back leg is straight, heel on the floor and toes of both feet facing straight ahead. Hold for 10 seconds, then repeat with the other leg.

Back of Upper Arm Stretch Stand with feet a comfortable distance apart and knees slightly bent. Raise one elbow and ease your hand down your back, using the other arm to assist. Hold for 10 seconds. Relax, and repeat with the other arm.

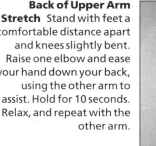

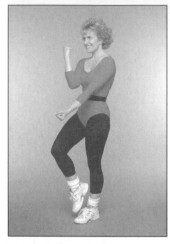

March on the spot, flexing and straightening alternate arms in front. Do 32.

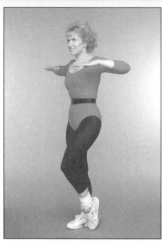

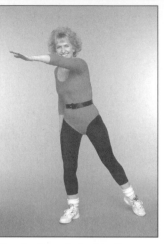

Walk on the spot, drawing your elbows backwards and forwards as you step. Do 32.

Touch alternate feet to the floor, reaching across with alternate arms. Do 32.

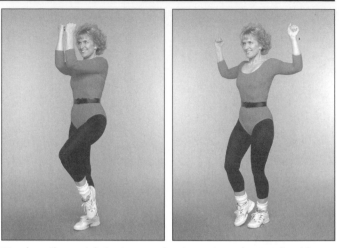

March on the spot, bringing your bent arms in and out at shoulder level. Do 32.

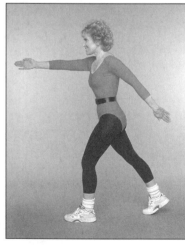

Touch the floor behind with one foot and swing the same arm forwards. Bring the foot back to the centre and repeat with the other leg and arm. Do 32 on alternate sides.

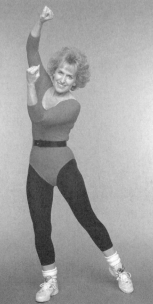

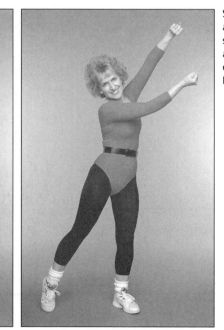

Step and touch alternate feet to the side, swinging your arms in a figure of eight as you step. Do 32.

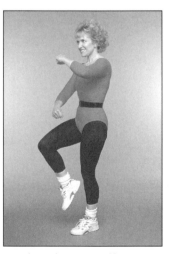

March on the spot and beat an imaginary drum with your hands. Do 32.

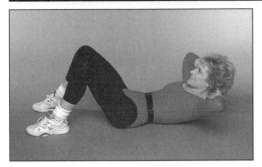 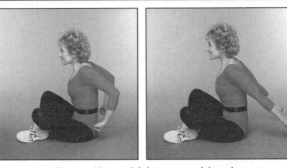 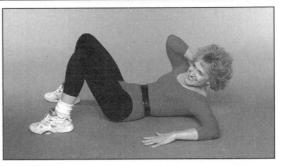

Tummy Toner Lie on your back with knees bent and your *tummy pulled in tightly*. Place your hands behind your neck and slowly raise your head and shoulders off the floor. Raise on a count of 2, then return to the floor on a count of 2. Do 16–18.

Upper Arm Toner Sit up with legs crossed, bend your arms and raise them behind you as high as possible. Keeping your elbows still, straighten your arms then bend them again. Do 16–18.

Waist Toner Lie on the floor with knees bent. Place one hand behind your head and have the other arm on the floor for support. Raise your head and shoulder and bring the elbow towards the opposite knee, taking care not to roll the hips. Return to the floor, and repeat. Do 16–18, then repeat to the other side.

Back Strengthener Lie face down with your hands placed on your seat. Slowly raise your chest and shoulders off the floor, using the muscles in your spine. Return to the floor, and repeat. Do 16–18.

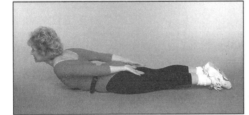 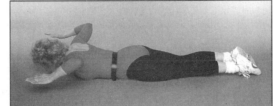

Upper Back Strengthener Lie face down with arms bent at shoulder level. Raise your arms, squeezing your shoulder blades together as much as possible. Lower your arms, and repeat. Do 16–18.

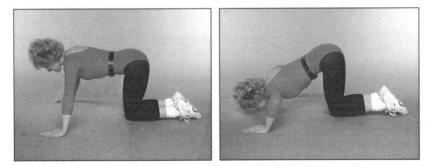 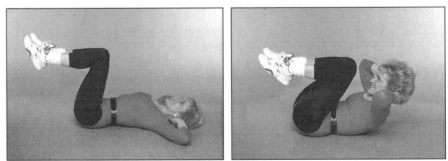

Chest Toner Position yourself on all fours with your hands placed on the floor slightly wider than shoulder-width apart. Slowly lower your head to the floor, then lift up again, keeping your chin in line with your hands. Keep your tummy tight and your back straight throughout. Repeat 16–18 times.

Tummy Streamliner Lie on your back with knees bent and raised over your hips, and place your hands on either side of your head. *Pull your tummy in tightly* and lift your head and shoulders and, at the same time, bring your knees in towards your chest. Return to the floor, and repeat. Do 16–18.

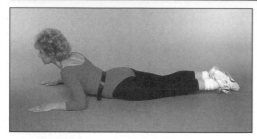

Tummy Stretch Lying face down, place your arms to the sides with elbows bent. Slowly raise your head and shoulders off the floor, supporting yourself on your forearms and elbows, and feel the stretch down the front of your abdomen. Hold for 10 seconds.

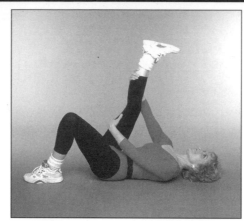

Back of Thigh Stretch Lie on your back with knees bent. Take hold of one leg and raise it, straightening it as far as is comfortable. Ease the leg towards you with your hands and hold for 10–15 seconds. Relax, and repeat with the other leg.

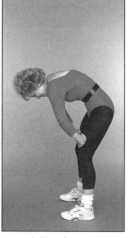

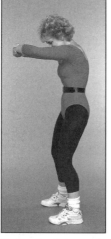

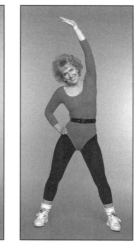

Back Stretch Standing with feet a comfortable distance apart, rest your hands on your thighs, just above your knees, to support your weight. Arch your back as much as possible, pulling your tummy in, and feel the stretch down your back. Hold for 10 seconds.

Upper Back Stretch Round your back and raise your arms in front to shoulder level to separate your shoulder blades. Hold for 10 seconds.

Chest Stretch Take your arms behind you and place one hand on top of the other. Raise your arms and feel the stretch across your chest. Hold for 10 seconds.

Back of Upper Arm Stretch Raise one elbow and ease your hand down your back, using the other arm to assist. Hold for 10 seconds. Relax, and repeat with the other arm.

Waist Stretch Place one hand on your thigh for support and lean to the side as you reach the opposite arm over. Hold for 10 seconds. Slowly straighten up, and repeat to the other side.

POSITIVE THOUGHT FOR THE DAY

Today, let's see how we can make good use of our time each day so that each day becomes a day of achievement. Maximising the productivity of your day is not a complicated matter but simply one that warrants some thought the evening before. Just before you leave your office or place of work, spend five minutes making a list of the jobs that need to be done the next day. Jot them down in no particular order. Next, go through that list and number them in the order of priority. The next morning, before you do any other job, look at your list and make sure that you start with the number one job. So often the most important job is the one we like least, but once we have done it the feeling of satisfaction and relief is nothing short of euphoric, so don't be frightened of tackling the worst jobs. Putting them off just causes stress. Doing them creates great satisfaction. Once you have finished the first job on your list, proceed to the second and the third and so on. If you go through your tasks in this fashion you will maximise the time that you have available. I know of no better way of achieving more in our everyday lives. Remember that saying 'people don't plan to fail but people do fail to plan'. If you are a planner and you are able to create some self-discipline in your daily life you will be absolutely staggered at what you can achieve.

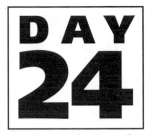

DAY 24

Are you feeling slimmer and fitter as each day arrives? Do you keep looking in the mirror? It's brilliant to see those inches disappearing, isn't it? Unfortunately, as the day proceeds, our abdomens seem to get bigger. This is not surprising – as we eat and drink our stomachs will inevitably fill up. This is why good posture is so important – it means we have to pull the abdomen in all day. However, if you are finding that your abdomen only becomes distended at certain times, this could be due to a food allergy. Some people find that if they drink coffee their stomach seems to blow up out of all proportion. If you suspect that you could have an allergy to one particular type of food, try eliminating the suspect food for three days, then re-introduce it and see if you have a reaction. Further help can be obtained through a nutritionist or dietary specialist. We often tend to find excuses for our shape by laying the blame on some physical abnormality. I am often amused by one gentleman who has been trying to persuade me that his distended paunch is due to the fact that he has a lot of muscle in that area. We only need to look at a body builder and see the form created by exaggerated muscle tone to realise that a big paunch has nothing to do with muscle but everything to do with fat. Eating a low-fat diet and taking regular exercise is the only way to get rid of the fat and tone up our muscles. Long-term success certainly can be achieved, but it does take some serious effort. So far you have proved you are capable of serious effort, and you now have only a few days before you complete this 28-day campaign. Enjoy today's menus, execute the exercises with precision and look forward to the end of the week. Be strong-willed, disciplined, energetic and enthusiastic, and you will be even slimmer by weighing and measuring day. Have a great day.

MENU

BREAKFAST

2 oz (50 g) Special K with milk from allowance
1 piece fresh fruit

or

1 wholemeal muffin or 1 bagel or 2 oz (50 g) toast, spread with 2 tsp jam or marmalade; 1 piece fresh fruit

LUNCH

P **Green Salad with Sesame Salad Dressing**
Mix 2 tsp reduced-oil salad dressing and 2 tsp low-fat natural yogurt with 1/2 tsp sesame seeds. Season with freshly ground black pepper. Spread on 2 slices wholemeal bread and fill with shredded lettuce, finely chopped celery, green pepper, watercress, spring onion and tomatoes

Q 8 oz (200 g) jacket potato topped with 4 oz (100 g) low-fat cottage cheese (plain or with chives or pineapple), plus salad

R **Chunky Vegetable Soup** (page 158)
plus 1 slice wholemeal bread (no butter)

DINNER

STARTER
Hot asparagus tips served with 1 tbsp reduced-oil salad dressing mixed with 1 tbsp low-fat natural yogurt

R **Tuna, Mushroom and Pasta Serenade** (page 169)

Q **Spaghetti Bolognese** (page 161)

V Batchelor's Beanfeast Mexican Chilli served with boiled rice (2 oz/50 g [dry weight] per person) or jacket potato, plus salad

DESSERT
Low-fat Rice Pudding (page 178)

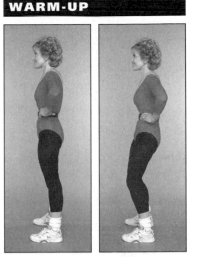

Stand in a good posture with your tummy in and your back straight, and tilt your pelvis forwards and upwards. Relax, and repeat. Do 8.

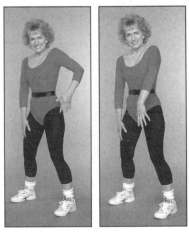

Roll alternate shoulders backwards, transferring your weight from one foot to the other. Do 16, then repeat, this time rolling shoulders forwards.

CONTINUED ▶

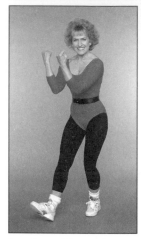

Step from side to side and tap the opposite heel on the floor in front, flexing and straightening your arms as you step. Do 16.

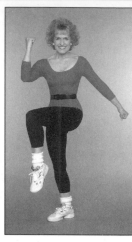

Raise alternate knees across and aim to touch with opposite elbow. Keep your tummy pulled in and your back straight. Do 16.

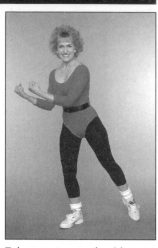

Take two steps to the side, making a scooping movement with your arms as if shovelling snow. Repeat to the other side. Do 16, alternating sides.

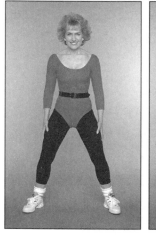

With feet a comfortable distance apart, transfer your weight from one foot to the other, bending your knees and tapping the toes of the opposite foot as you step. Do 16.

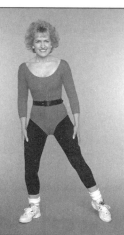

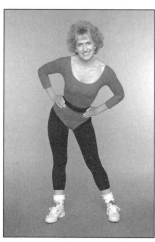

Rotate your hips in a clockwise direction. Do 8, then repeat in an anti-clockwise direction.

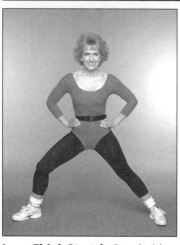

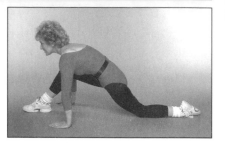

Upper Thigh Stretch Kneeling as shown, take your weight on to your front foot. Ease your hips forwards and feel the stretch in the front thigh of the back leg. Hold for 10 seconds, then relax, and repeat with the other leg

Inner Thigh Stretch Stand with feet wide apart and bend one knee over the ankle. The other leg is straight with toes facing forwards, and your hips are square. Feel the stretch in the inner thigh of the straight leg and hold for 10 seconds. Relax, and repeat on the other side.

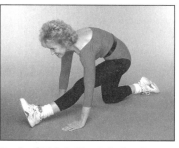

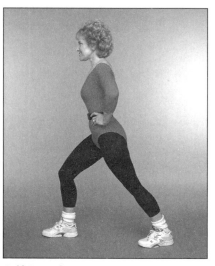

Back of Thigh Stretch Resting on one knee, extend the other leg forwards and take your weight on to your hands placed at either side of your front leg. Ease your seat back towards your heel, but don't sit on it. Feel the stretch at the back of the front leg, and hold for 10 seconds. Relax, then change legs, and repeat.

Calf Stretch Stand with one leg in front of the other and bend the front knee. The toes of both feet are facing forwards, and the back heel is down. Keep your weight slightly forwards and feel the stretch in the calf muscle of your back leg. Hold for 10 seconds, then change legs and repeat.

Step and lunge to one side, reaching across with opposite arm. Only the toes of the straight leg should touch the floor. Try to straighten the arm and leg as much as possible as you lunge. Repeat to the other side. Do 32 to alternate sides.

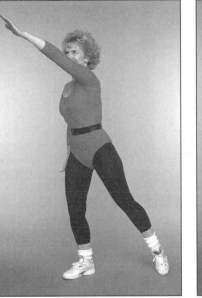

Step to the side and curtsey with one leg behind, swinging your arms out to the side and crossing them in front as you step. Do 32.

Step to one side and curtsey, swinging your arms out and in to cross high above your head. Do 32.

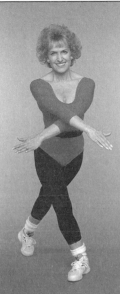

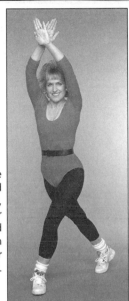

Jog on the spot, flexing and straightening alternate arms in front. Keep your knees soft and bring your heels down as you land. Do 32.

Extend alternate legs out to the side, clapping your hands overhead. Do 32.

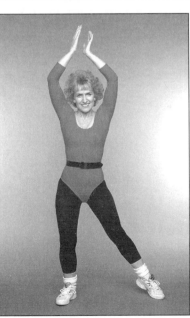

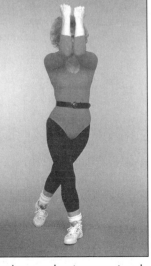

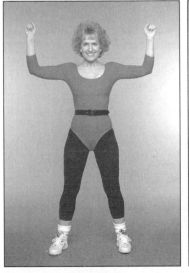

Step and curtsey with alternate legs, bringing your bent arms out and in at shoulder level. Do 32.

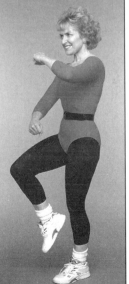

March on the spot and beat an imaginary drum with your hands. Do 32.

Upper Arm Toner
Standing with feet a comfortable distance apart and knees slightly bent, bend your arms and raise your elbows as high as possible behind you. Straighten your arms behind you, then bend them again. Repeat 16–18 times, keeping the elbows as high as possible throughout.

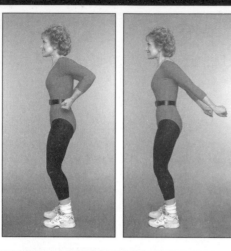

Outer Thigh Toner
Lying with both knees slightly bent, dip the knee of the top leg on the floor in front and then, leading with the heel, extend and straighten it towards the corner of the room. Repeat this dipping and straightening movement 16–18 times, ensuring the hips remain square. Roll over, and repeat with the other leg.

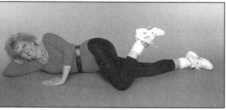

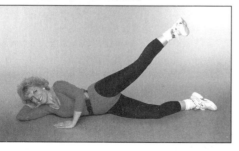

Inner Thigh Toner Bend the top leg and rest it on the floor, in front of your hips. Keeping the bottom leg straight, lift it up and down 16–18 times. Roll over, and repeat with the other leg.

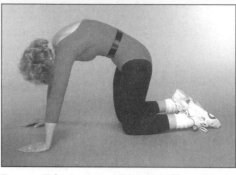

Tummy Trimmer Position yourself on all fours and pull your tummy muscles in as tightly as you can to arch your spine. Relax, and repeat 16–18 times.

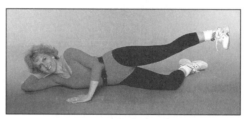

Outer Thigh Toner Lie on your side with your bottom leg bent and your top leg straight. Raise the top leg, keeping your hips square and your toes aiming slightly downwards. Do not raise the leg too high. Lower, then repeat. Do 16–18, then roll over and repeat with the other leg.

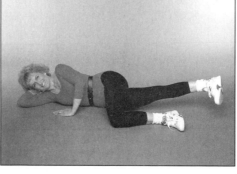

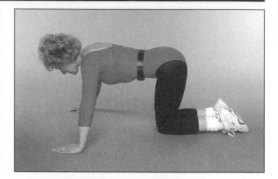

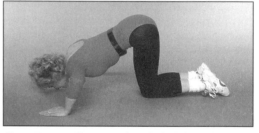

Chest Toner Place your hands slightly wider than shoulder-width apart. Slowly lower your head to the floor, then lift up again, keeping your chin in line with your hands. Keep your tummy tight and your back straight throughout. Repeat 16–18 times.

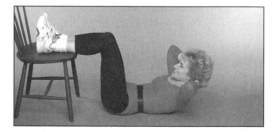

Tummy Toner Lie on your back with your feet placed against a wall or on a sturdy chair, and support your neck with your hands. *Pulling your tummy in tightly*, raise your head and shoulders off the floor, keeping a distance between your chin and your chest. Raise on a count of 2, and return to the floor on a count of 2. Repeat 16–18 times.

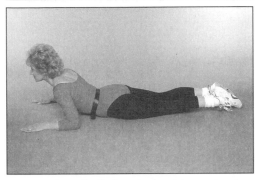

Tummy Stretch Lie face down with arms bent. Slowly raise your head and shoulders off the floor, supporting yourself on your forearms and elbows, and feel the stretch down the front of your abdomen. Hold for 10 seconds.

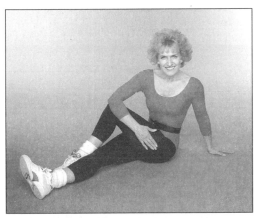

Outer Thigh Stretch Sit up with one leg extended and the other leg bent and placed across the straight leg approximately level with the knee. Use the opposite elbow to ease the bent knee across. Hold for 10 seconds. Relax, and change position to repeat with the other leg.

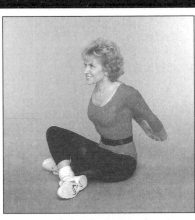

Chest Stretch Sitting with legs crossed, raise your arms and clasp your hands behind your back to stretch the muscles across your chest. Hold for 10 seconds.

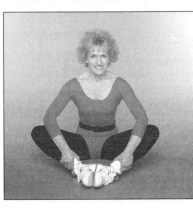

Back of Upper Arm Stretch Raise one elbow and ease your hand down your back. Use the other arm to ease it further. Hold for 10 seconds. Repeat with the other arm.

Inner Thigh Stretch Sit up with knees bent and soles of the feet together. Using your elbows, gently ease your knees down as far as is comfortable. Hold for 15 seconds.

POSITIVE THOUGHT FOR THE DAY

In our daily lives we waste so much time thinking about unimportant issues and worrying about situations over which we have no control. Try to be effective with the use of your time and put 'pockets' of time to maximum use. Collecting the groceries on your way back from the office is a good way to save on journey time. Use gaps between appointments to make short telephone calls and answer messages. Don't put off any jobs that you could do now. Replying to an enquiry promptly not only impresses the caller, but it also enables you to clear it out of your mind. If you have a message on your desk to ring someone and you keep putting it off, this leaves you with a tremendous time-wasting situation as you keep picking the message up and deciding yet again 'Oh, I'll leave that for now'. Whatever the problem, it is so much better to resolve it instantly and get all the negative and worry feelings out of the way so that you can proceed positively with the next job in hand.

The same applies to replying to business letters. I try never to read a letter twice. It is a waste of time to pick up the same letter and read it three times only to decide that it can be replied to later as it is non-urgent. It's all about self-discipline and using your time to the very best effect.

You only have four days to go on this diet and exercise programme. Give it your very best effort. Have willpower as strong as iron and be physically active as if your life depended on it. The rewards from achieving this enormous goal at the end of 28 days will be wonderful. Just go for it.

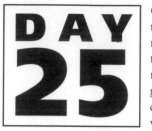

DAY 25

Only four days to go and you need to concentrate wholly on reaching your goal. As you continue to lose weight you will almost inevitably experience hunger pangs from time to time. It may be tempting to have a snack mid-morning or mid-afternoon, but once you become accustomed to such indulgences, the occasional treat becomes a full-time habit – a habit that has to be broken. If you feel hungry it takes real mental discipline to programme yourself not to eat anything until the next mealtime, but once the message has got through you can turn your mind to something else and the stomach rumblings will mostly disappear. Conditioning yourself to ignore hunger pangs is well worth the commitment.

Today's exercises are more challenging than any you have done so far. The menus should stimulate your palate and make you feel rewarded, not deprived. Try to be as physically active as possible today as you go about your everyday work and look forward to feeling even slimmer tomorrow.

MENU

BREAKFAST

4 fl oz (100 ml) orange juice; 1 wholemeal roll (2 oz/50 g) spread with 2 tsp honey, marmalade or jam; 1 x 5 oz (125 g) diet yogurt

or

1/4 pint/5 fl oz (125 ml) orange juice
4 brown Ryvitas spread with Marmite and topped with 4 oz (100 g) low-fat cottage cheese

LUNCH

P Tuna, Cucumber and Watercress Open Sandwich
Spread 2 slices wholemeal bread with reduced-oil salad dressing.
Mix 1/2 bunch chopped watercress leaves with 2 tbsp reduced-oil salad dressing and a little lemon juice. Add 2 oz (50 g) tuna. Spread on the bread, garnish with watercress and cucumber and serve as an open sandwich

Q Crunchy Salad with Chicken and French Bread
Mix 100 g (4 oz) bean sprouts with 1 dessert apple, chopped,
1 tbsp raisins and 1 small tin mandarin oranges. Serve with 2 oz (50 g)
chopped chicken and 1 oz (25 g) French bread
4 oz (100 g) grapes

R Cream of Leek and Potato Soup (page 158)
plus 1 slice wholemeal bread (no butter)

DINNER

STARTER
Mussels in White Wine (page 157)
R Cullercoats Pie (page 168)
Q Tuna Salsa
Allow 6 oz (150 g) tuna per person. Heat contents of 1 x 16 oz (400 g)
jar of Colman's Tuna Salsa Sauce (serves 4) in a saucepan for 2–3 minutes,
stirring occasionally. Add the tuna, stir gently until hot.
Serve with boiled brown rice (2 oz/50 g [dry weight] per person)

V Batchelor's Beanfeast Bolognese-style Soya in Rich Tomato Sauce, served with
egg-free spaghetti (2 oz/50 g [dry weight] per person)

DESSERT
Prune Cake (page 178)

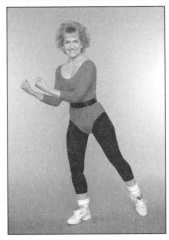

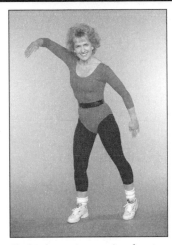

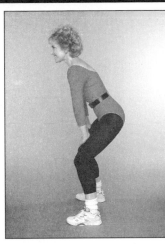

Take two steps to the side, making a scooping movement with your arms as if shovelling snow. Repeat to the other side. Do 16, alternating sides.

Circle alternate arms in a front crawl swimming motion, transferring your weight from one foot to the other. Do 16.

With feet wide apart, bend your knees and squat down. Make sure your knees bend over the ankles. Come up again, and repeat. Do 8.

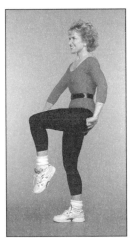

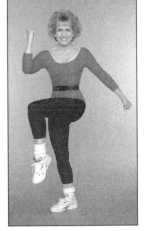

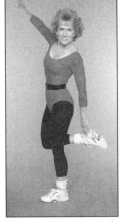

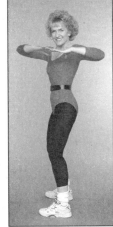

Raise alternate knees in front, pressing down with both arms. Keep your tummy tight and back straight. Do 16.

Raise alternate knees and aim to touch with opposite elbow. Do 16.

Raise alternate ankles behind and touch with opposite hands. Do 32.

Keeping your hips square, twist your upper body from side to side. Do not jerk. Do 8 to each side.

Back Stretch Standing with feet a comfortable distance apart, rest your hands on your thighs, just above your knees, to support your weight. Arch your back as much as possible, pulling your tummy in, and feel the stretch down your back. Hold for 10 seconds.

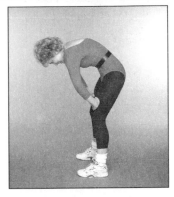

Back of Thigh Stretch Bend one knee and, keeping your weight on that foot, extend the other leg in front, toes raised. Feel the stretch at the back of the knee and the thigh. Hold for 10 seconds, then change legs and repeat.

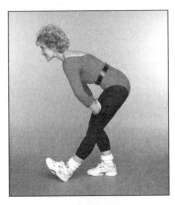

Calf Stretch Shift your weight on to the front leg and bend the knee. Your back leg is straight, heel on the floor and toes of both feet facing straight ahead. Keep your weight slightly forwards and feel the stretch in the calf muscle of your back leg. Hold for 10 seconds, then change legs and repeat.

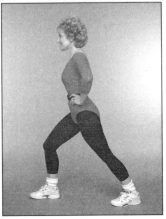

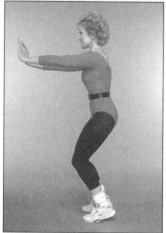

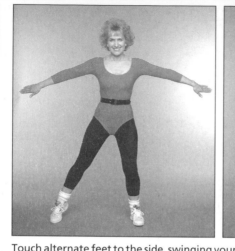

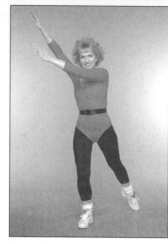

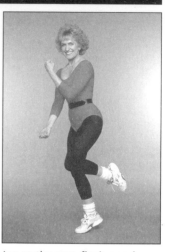

With feet close together, alternately bend and straighten your knees, swinging your arms forwards and backwards. Do 32.

Touch alternate feet to the side, swinging your arms out and in and crossing them in front as you bring the leg in. Do 32.

Step with one foot and touch the other foot to the floor behind on a diagonal, swinging your arms high to the side. Repeat to the other side. Do 24.

Jog on the spot, flexing and straightening alternate arms. Make sure your knees are soft and heels are down as you land. Do 32.

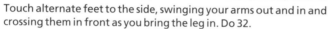

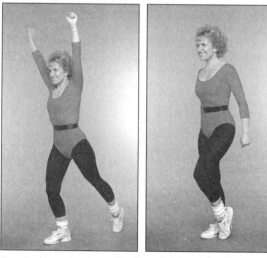

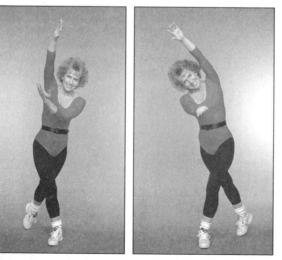

Stand with knees together, feet facing straight ahead and arms stretched above your head. Ski down, bending your knees and swinging your arms down and to the back of you. Return to the starting position, and repeat, keeping your chest lifted throughout. Do 32.

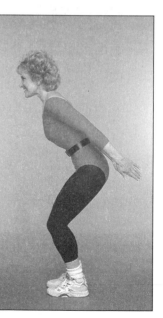

Touch alternate feet to the floor behind, raising your arms above your head as you touch behind and then lowering them as you bring the leg in. Do 32.

With feet apart, step from side to side and touch alternate feet behind, creating a figure of eight with your arms as you step. Do 32.

Bottom Toner
Hold on to the back of a chair and raise one leg behind you, keeping the leg straight and squeezing your seat as you raise. Lower the leg, and repeat. Keep your tummy tight, hips square and your back straight throughout. Do 16–18, then repeat with the other leg.

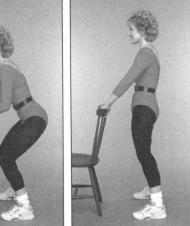

Bottom Streamliner Place your feet a comfortable distance apart, with your toes and knees facing slightly outwards. Bend your knees as if you were going to sit on a chair behind you, then straighten your knees and push your pelvis forwards, squeezing your buttocks together. Repeat 16–18 times.

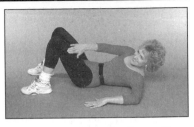

Waist Toner Lie on the floor with knees bent. Supporting yourself with one arm, reach across your body with the other arm, pressing your tummy down as you reach. Take care not to roll the hips. Return to the floor, and repeat. Do 16–18, then repeat to the other side.

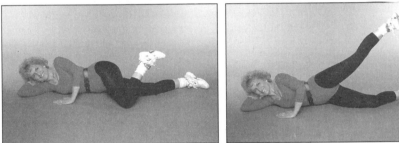

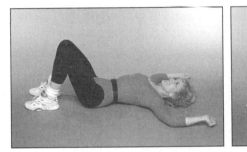

Outer Thigh Toner Lie on your side with both knees slightly bent. Dip the knee of the top leg on the floor in front and then, leading with the heel, extend and straighten it towards the corner of the room. Repeat this dipping and straightening movement 16–18 times, ensuring the hips remain square. Roll over, and repeat with the other leg.

Tummy and Chest Toner Lie on your back with knees bent and arms bent at shoulder level. *Pulling your tummy in tightly*, raise your head and shoulders off the floor and at the same time squeeze your elbows together. Return to the floor, and repeat. Do 16–18.

Bottom Toner Resting your weight on your forearms, extend one leg behind you. Keeping the leg straight, raise it in line with your hips – no higher – then lower it again. Raise and lower the leg 16–18 times, keeping your tummy in and your back flat throughout. Repeat with the other leg.

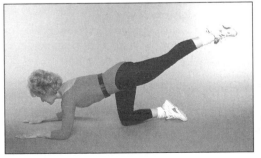

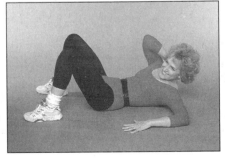

Waist Toner Lying on your back with both knees bent, place one hand behind your neck and have the other arm on the floor for support. Raise your head and shoulder and bring your elbow towards the opposite knee, taking care not to roll your hips. Return to the floor, and repeat. Do 16–18, then repeat to the other side.

CONTINUED ▶

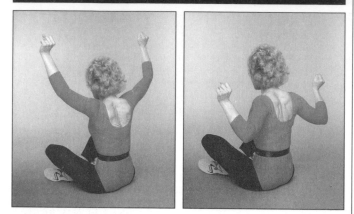

Upper Back Toner Sit upright with your legs crossed. Take your arms above your head and reach up. Now pull the elbows back and down to squeeze your shoulder blades together. Raise the arms again, and repeat. Do 16–18.

Tummy Streamliner Lie on your back with knees bent and raised over your hips, and place your hands on either side of your head. *Pull your tummy in tightly* and lift your head and shoulders and, at the same time, bring your knees in towards your chest. Return to the floor and repeat. Do 16–18.

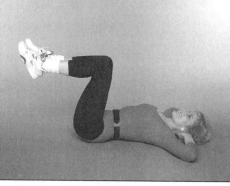

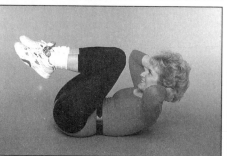

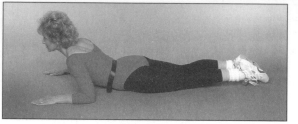

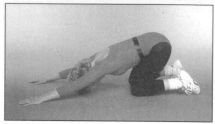

Tummy Stretch Lying face down, place your arms to the sides with elbows bent. Slowly raise your head and shoulders off the floor, supporting yourself on your forearms and elbows, and feel the stretch down the front of your abdomen. Hold for 10 seconds.

Seat Stretch Start in the all fours position. Slowly ease your hips backwards without touching your heels and, at the same time, extend your arms in front. Hold for 10 seconds.

Waist and Outer Thigh Stretch Sit up straight with one leg extended and the other leg placed across it. Slowly twist your body away from the bent knee, using the opposite elbow to ease the bent knee further across. Hold for 10 seconds, then change legs and repeat to the other side.

POSITIVE THOUGHT FOR THE DAY

Only three more days to go now. Do you notice any changes in the way you think as well as how you look? Can you feel that extra confidence emerging and growing? However, be aware that people are only too happy to put labels on each and every one of us – comments like 'you'll never be slim, you weren't made that way' or 'you don't like exercise, do you?' Yet all these labels that people are only too ready to give us are ones that we so often give ourselves. The more we label ourselves as having a particular weakness, the greater our chances of failure. So turn these negatives into positives and start programming your brain into a positive attitude. Start saying, 'I'm good at following this diet, it's easy.' 'I am really enjoying these exercises because they are within my capability and I can feel the good they are doing,' or 'I know this diet is working because I feel healthy and so much slimmer.' We *do* need to keep reminding ourselves. Getting into the right frame of mind is important in our quest for success. Throw away the labels, throw away the barriers, be positive and look forward to whatever *you* want to achieve. If you want it badly enough, you'll get it.

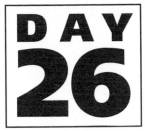

DAY 26

For those of us who enjoy food – and the very fact that we have to watch our weight is proof that we do – it is important to make each mealtime an occasion. Always sit down to eat and never eat on the move. Never read at the table even if you are on your own. Instead, savour every mouthful and make each meal a feast. Use attractive dishes and set the table properly so that you feel you're at a banquet. Always have some extra fillers available in the form of a ready-prepared salad in a yogurt and garlic dressing or some extra cooked vegetables. Have sparkling water or a low-calorie drink to hand to help fill you up. Look around the local supermarkets for new and interesting foods and experiment with different flavours. For salads, don't just use lettuce, tomato and cucumber, but include other salad ingredients such as different types of lettuce, watercress, spring onions, chives, carrots, and beetroot – all kinds of lovely, nutritious foods which can help fill you up yet which cost very little in calories. Keep a selection of low-fat dressings to hand to use on salads or spread on bread when making sandwiches. Don't just have a plain ham or chicken sandwich. Fill it with salad and vegetables. Take these suggestions on board in the long term and make them part of your future eating habits.

After today there are only two more days to the end of this 28-day plan. Make a huge effort to be as physically active as possible, don't cheat, and enjoy the meals that have been designed for you. Remember your posture and hold that tummy in as much as you possibly can throughout the day. Have a good one.

MENU

BREAKFAST

3 apricots soaked overnight in herbal or regular tea and served with 5 fl oz (175 g) diet yogurt or low-fat fromage frais

or

3 fl oz (75 ml) orange juice
6 oz (150 g) chopped melon mixed with 1 oz (25 g) All-Bran and topped with 2 fl oz (50 ml) milk (in addition to allowance)

LUNCH

P *Cottage Cheese and Sweetcorn Roll*
Mix 1 finely sliced spring onion with 1 heaped tbsp low-fat cottage cheese and 2 oz (50 g) sweetcorn. Spread a crusty roll or French stick (2 oz/50 g) with reduced-oil salad dressing and fill with the cottage cheese mixture

Q *Fruit Compote*
4 oz (100 g) melon, chopped, mixed, with segments of 1 small orange or satsuma and 2 oz (50 g) pineapple (canned in natural juice), topped with 1 x 8 oz (200 g) pot Müllerlight yogurt

R *Tuna Pasta with Tomatoes* (page 169)

DINNER

STARTER
Chicken and Sweetcorn Soup (page 158)
R *Tarragon Chicken Salad* (page 166)

Q 8 oz (200 g) any white fish, steamed, poached or microwaved, served with unlimited vegetables and parsley sauce (made without fat) or tomato sauce

V Asda World Bistro Vegetable Chilli (392 g can serves 1) with boiled brown rice (2 oz/50 g) [dry weight] per person) and salad

DESSERT
Fruit Sundae (page 177)

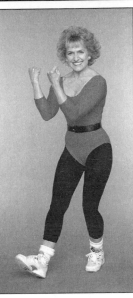

Step from side to side and tap the opposite heel on the floor in front, flexing and straightening your arms as you step. Do 16.

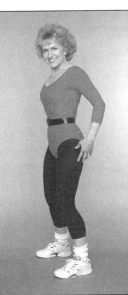

Roll both shoulders backwards while transferring your weight from one foot to the other. Do 16.

CONTINUED ▶

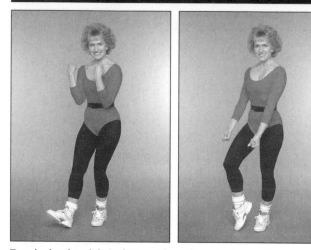

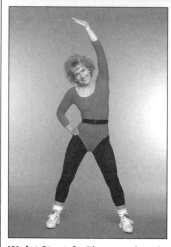

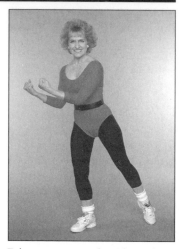

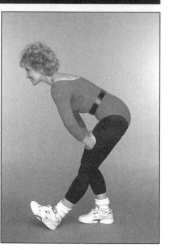

Tap the heel and then the toe of one foot, flexing and straightening both arms. Do 8, then repeat with the other foot.

Take two steps to the side, making a scooping movement with your arms as if shovelling snow. Repeat to the other side. Do 16, alternating sides.

Waist Stretch Place one hand on your thigh for support and lean to the side as you reach the opposite arm over. Hold for 10 seconds. Slowly straighten up, and repeat to the other side.

Back of Thigh Stretch Bend one knee and, keeping your weight on that foot, extend the other leg in front, toes raised. Feel the stretch at the back of the knee and the thigh. Hold for 10 seconds, then change legs and repeat.

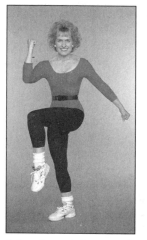

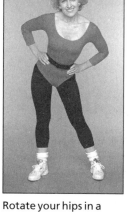

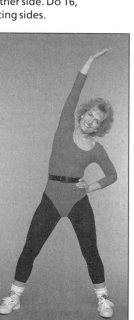

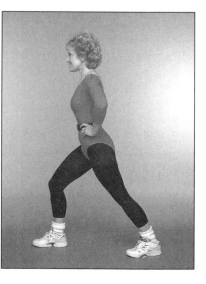

Stand with feet a comfortable distance apart, one arm raised with palm facing upwards, the other hand on your hip. Lean directly to the side, reaching over with the raised arm. Do not twist the hips. Return to the starting position, and repeat to the other side. Do 12 to each side.

Calf Stretch Shift your weight on to the front leg and bend the knee. Your back leg is straight, heel on the floor and toes of both feet facing straight ahead. Keep your weight slightly forwards and feel the stretch in the calf muscle of your back leg. Hold for 10 seconds, then change legs and repeat.

Raise alternate knees and aim to touch with opposite elbow. Do 16.

Rotate your hips in a clockwise direction. Do 8, then repeat in an anti-clockwise direction.

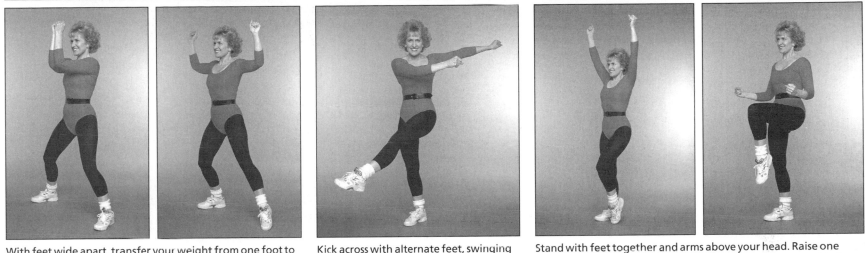

With feet wide apart, transfer your weight from one foot to the other, opening and closing your bent arms at shoulder level as you step. Do 32.

Kick across with alternate feet, swinging your arms from side to side in the opposite direction to your feet. Do 32.

Stand with feet together and arms above your head. Raise one knee twice, each time bringing your arms down. Repeat with the other knee. Do 32 double knee raises and arm pulleys, keeping your tummy tight throughout.

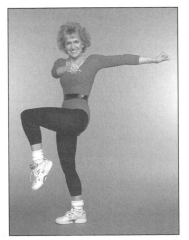 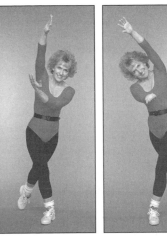 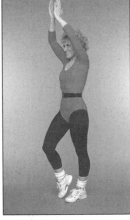 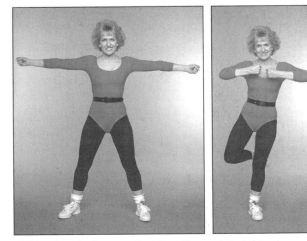

Keeping your tummy pulled in throughout, raise alternate knees across your body, swinging your arms from side to side. Do 32.

With feet apart, step from side to side and touch alternate feet behind, creating a figure of eight with your arms as you step. Do 32.

March on the spot, clapping your hands above your head. Do 32.

Kick back with alternate feet, bending and straightening your arms in front. Do 32.

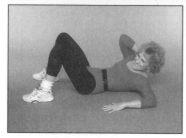

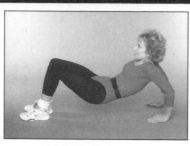

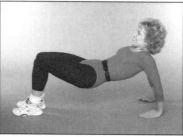

Waist Toner Lie on your back with knees bent. Place one hand behind your neck and have the other arm on the floor for support. Raise the head and shoulder and bring your elbow towards the opposite knee, taking care not to roll your hips. Return to the floor, and repeat. Do 16–18, then repeat to the other side.

Upper Arm Toner Place your arms behind you with fingers facing forwards, and lift your hips off the floor so that your weight is supported by your feet and your hands. Now, straighten your arms to raise your hips further and try to straighten your body as much as possible. Lower your hips without returning completely to the floor. Continue to raise and lower your body, and repeat as many times as possible. As this is an advanced exercise, start off with one or two and gradually increase the number of repetitions as you become stronger.

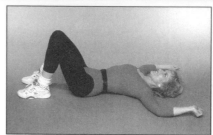

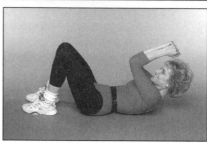

Tummy and Chest Toner Lie back with knees bent and arms bent at shoulder level. *Pulling your tummy in tightly*, raise your head and shoulders off the floor and at the same time squeeze your elbows together. Return to the floor, and repeat. Do 16–18.

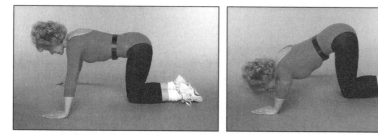

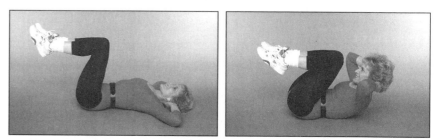

Chest Toner Position yourself on all fours, placing your hands slightly wider than shoulder-width apart. Slowly lower your head to the floor, then lift up again, keeping your chin in line with your hands. Keep your tummy tight and your back straight throughout. Repeat 16–18 times.

Tummy Streamliner Lie on your back with knees bent and raised over your hips, and place your hands on either side of your head. *Pull your tummy in tightly* and lift your head and shoulders and, at the same time, bring your knees in towards your chest. Return to the floor, and repeat. Do 16–18.

Back Strengthener Lie face down with your hands placed on your seat. Slowly raise your chest and shoulders off the floor, using the muscles in your spine. Return to the floor, and repeat. Do 16–18.

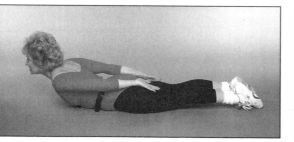

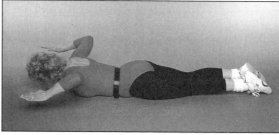

Upper Back Strengthener Place your arms to the sides with elbows bent at shoulder level. Raise your arms, squeezing your shoulder blades together as much as possible. Lower your arms, and repeat. Do 16–18.

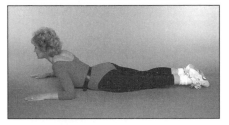

Tummy Stretch Still lying face down with arms bent, slowly raise your head and shoulders off the floor, supporting yourself on your forearms and elbows, and feel the stretch down the front of your abdomen. Hold for 10 seconds.

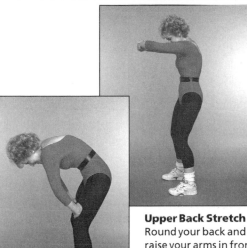

Back Stretch Standing with feet a comfortable distance apart, rest your hands on your thighs, just above your knees, to support your weight. Arch your back as much as possible, pulling your tummy in, and feel the stretch down your back. Hold for 10 seconds.

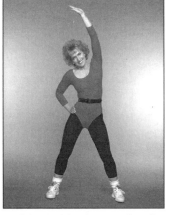

Upper Back Stretch Round your back and raise your arms in front to shoulder level to separate your shoulder blades. Hold for 10 seconds.

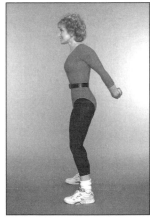

Chest Stretch Take your arms behind you and place one hand on top of the other. Raise your arms and feel the stretch across your chest. Hold for 10 seconds.

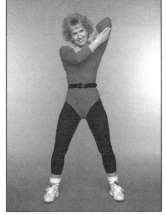

Back of Upper Arm Stretch Raise one elbow and ease your hand down your back, using the other arm to assist. Hold for 10 seconds. Relax, and repeat with the other arm.

Waist Stretch Place one hand on your thigh for support and lean to the side as you reach the opposite arm over. Hold for 10 seconds. Slowly straighten up, and repeat to the other side.

POSITIVE THOUGHT FOR THE DAY

Whatever it is we undertake in life, we must avoid making excuses for past failures. I get really frustrated if a potential slimmer says to me, 'But I have always been big. I've always been over 12 stone (87 kg), so the chances of me getting down to nine stone (65.3 kg) are virtually zero.' Well, she certainly wasn't 12 stone (87 kg) when she was born, so obviously over a period of years the weight *has* been brought on by over-indulgence.

When we feel we are failing at something it's so easy to say, 'Well, I can't help it.' But we *can* help it. If you decide that you are going to give up a bad habit from now on, keep repeating to yourself that you've given it up, and you will. Rediscover the joys of doing what you know you *should* be doing instead and soon this becomes a habit. Bad habits need to be broken, and good habits must take their place.

Success is not something that happens automatically. We have to work at it. If you stick with this diet until you reach your goal weight, you will have been incredibly successful. Some people think to be successful you need to learn a skill or have a huge amount of knowledge. Certainly having an understanding of how things work will help, but 85 per cent of success is achieved through self-discipline, having the right attitude and building a confident self-image. Only around 15 per cent is actually down to skill and knowledge. You don't need to have a *huge* knowledge of how this diet works or what these exercises are doing for you. A basic knowledge is essential but the main ingredient is, without doubt, having the willpower and the right attitude and believing in yourself.

By the time you reach the end of this 28-day plan, or whenever you feel you have reached your ideal weight, all you have to do is to maintain your new-found confidence. You will then be at a stage where you can really turn your entire life around. If you take on board the various points that I have included in the positive thoughts each day, they will sow the seeds that will enable you to turn your life into a challenging and successful experience which will not only benefit you but also the rest of your family. Don't underestimate their value.

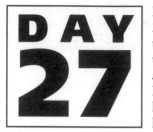

DAY 27

Here we are on Day 27 and it's time to try on the skirt or trousers again. Just *see* the difference! Isn't it incredible how many inches have disappeared from around your tummy? Would you have believed that you could lose that many in just four weeks? Having your measuring garment is a real reminder of what you have achieved. Somehow, by just using a tape measure and popping on the scales we don't really appreciate the progress we have actually made. Use that garment as a constant reminder of your success and don't ever let yourself fill it out again.

It is important that we do not become paranoid about our weight or fitness. To do so can be just as unhealthy as being overweight and unfit. We need to keep a sense of perspective and *not* let it rule our lives. Don't become a diet and fitness bore. The fact that you have achieved success on this programme doesn't mean that you shouldn't sympathise with those who perhaps have not been as fortunate and try to encourage them.

Try to play a game of sport tonight or participate in some physical activity after your evening meal, perhaps going dancing or swimming or taking a brisk walk. Work off your evening meal and prepare yourself for your last day tomorrow. Enjoy the meals and the exercises and really feel the benefit. Just one more day to go …

MENU

BREAKFAST

4 fl oz (100 ml) orange juice; $^3/_4$ oz (18.5 g) All-Bran with milk from allowance and 1 tsp sugar
1 oz (25 g) wholemeal toast with 2 tsp marmalade

or

3 fl oz (75 ml) orange juice; 1 oz (25 g) any bran cereal mixed with 5 oz (125 g) low-fat diet yogurt and 1 chopped fresh pear (including the skin)

LUNCH

ⓟ Turkey and Ham Pitta

1 wholemeal pitta filled with 1 oz (25 g) sliced cold cooked turkey, 1 oz (25 g) chopped ham, sliced tomato, peppers and 2 tbsp low-fat fromage frais, all mixed with reduced-oil salad dressing. Add a squeeze of lemon juice if you wish

ⓠ 8 oz (200 g) jacket potato topped with 4 oz (173 g) baked beans mixed with $^1/_4$ tsp chilli powder, plus salad

ⓡ Vegetable Crunch (page 173)

DINNER

STARTER
Prawn Cocktail
2 oz (50 g) prawns on a bed of shredded lettuce, topped with Prawn Cocktail Sauce (page 179)

ⓡ Cod, Bacon, Cheese and Onion Bake (page 167)

ⓠ Beef Casserole (page 161)

ⓥ 1 x 16 oz (400 g) can Heinz Lentil Whole Soup, plus 1 wholemeal roll (2 oz/50 g); 8 oz (200 g) jacket potato filled with 2 oz (50 g) sweetcorn, 2 oz (50 g) red kidney beans, 1 oz (25 g) raisins mixed with low-fat fromage frais or yogurt dressing, plus salad

DESSERT
Apricot and Banana Fool (page 176)

Roll both shoulders backwards while transferring your weight from one foot to the other. Do 16.

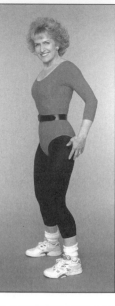

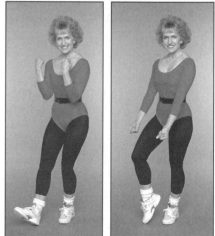

Tap the heel and then the toe of one foot, flexing and straightening both arms. Do 8, then repeat with the other foot.

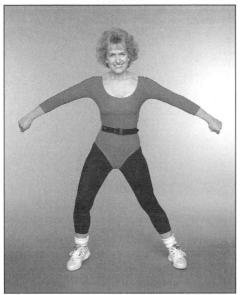

Take two steps to the side, swinging arms in and out as you step. Repeat to the other side. Do 16 to alternate sides.

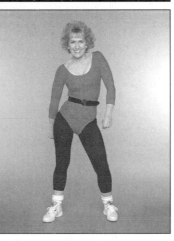

With feet a comfortable distance apart, raise one hip and at the same time raise the opposite shoulder. Repeat with the other hip and shoulder. Do 16 on alternate sides.

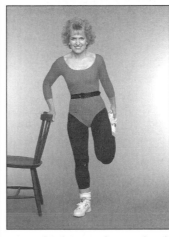

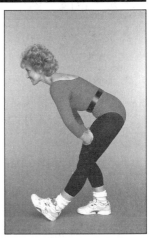

Front Thigh Stretch Stand and hold on to the back of a chair. Keeping your inside leg slightly bent, bend the other leg and take hold of your foot. Ease the foot back and up, keeping both knees aligned. Hold for 10 seconds. Release, then turn round and repeat with the other leg.

Back of Thigh Stretch
Bend one knee and, keeping your weight on that foot, extend the other leg in front, toes raised. Feel the stretch at the back of the knee and the thigh. Hold for 10 seconds, then change legs and repeat.

Calf Stretch Shift your weight on to the front leg and bend the knee. Your back leg is straight, heel on the floor and toes of both feet facing straight ahead. Keep your weight slightly forwards and feel the stretch in the calf muscle of your back leg. Hold for 10 seconds, then change legs and repeat.

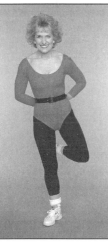

Kick back with alternate feet. Do 16.

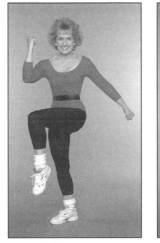

Raise alternate knees and aim to touch with opposite elbow. Do 16.

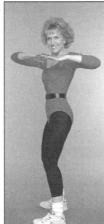

Standing with feet apart, reach over to the side. Repeat to the other side. Do 12 to each side.

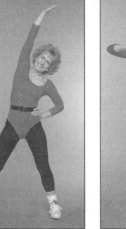

Keeping your hips square, twist your upper body from side to side. Do not jerk. Do 8 to each side.

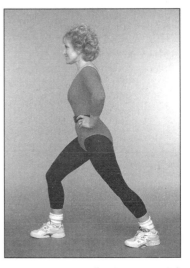

With feet wide apart, lunge from side to side, pressing the opposite arm across your body. Exert as much pressure as possible with each arm as you move from side to side. Do 32.

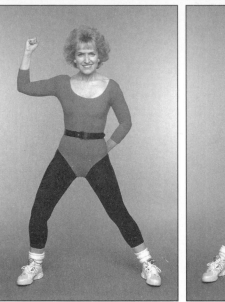

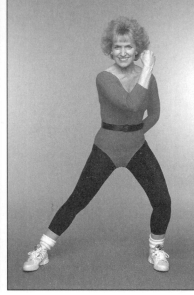

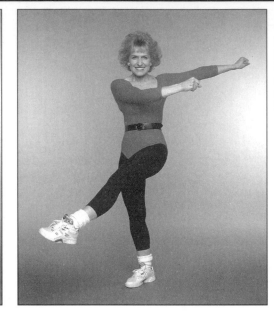

Kick across with alternate feet, swinging your arms from side to side in the opposite direction to your feet. Do 32.

Stand with feet together and arms above your head. Raise one knee twice, each time bringing your arms down. Repeat with the other knee. Do 16 double knee raises and arm pulleys, keeping your tummy tight throughout.

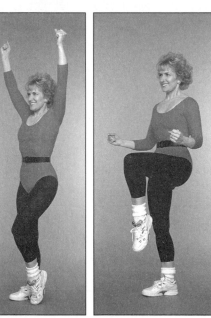

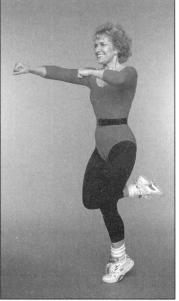

Jog on the spot, kicking your feet high to the back of you and punching your arms in front. Keep your knees soft and bring your heels down as you land. Do 32.

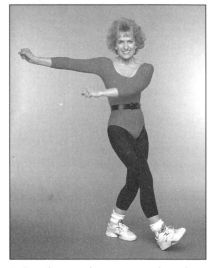

Swing alternate legs across and tap the floor with your heels, swinging your arms from side to side as you step. Do 16.

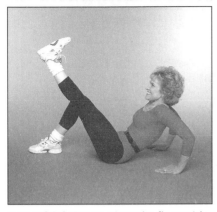

Front Thigh Toner Sit on the floor with both legs bent, and support your weight on your hands. Straighten one leg and raise it to the level of the other knee, then lower it again. Do 16–18 straight leg lifts, keeping your tummy tight. Repeat with the other leg.

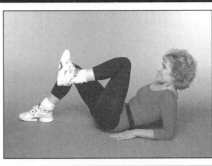
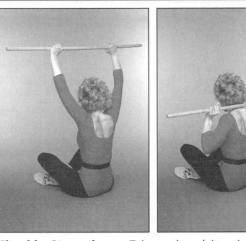

Shoulder Strengthener Take a pole and sit upright in a comfortable position. Raise the pole above your head, then lower it, squeezing your shoulder blades together. Repeat. Do 16–18, concentrating on bringing your shoulder blades together as you lower the pole.

Front Thigh Toner Supporting yourself on your arms, bend both knees. Bring one knee in towards your chest and then extend the leg straight out in front. Keep your tummy tight to support your back. Bring the leg towards your chest again, and repeat. Do 16–18, then repeat with the other leg.

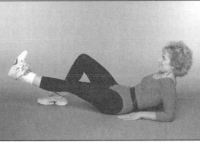

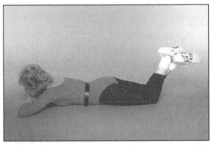

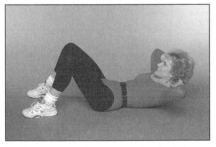

Tummy Toner Lie on your back with knees bent and your *tummy pulled in tightly*. Place your hands behind your neck and slowly raise your head and shoulders off the floor. Raise on a count of 2, then return to the floor on a count of 2. Do 16–18.

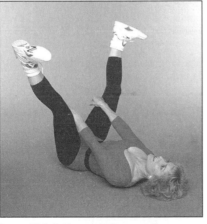

Inner Thigh Toner Raise your feet above your hips with legs apart, and place your hands on the inside of your thighs. Use your hands for resistance as you aim to bring your legs together. Keep your back pressed into the floor. Do 16–18.

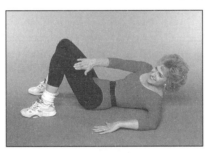

Waist Toner Bend your knees and place your feet on the floor. Supporting yourself with one arm, reach across your body with the other arm, pressing your tummy down as you reach. Take care not to roll the hips. Return to the floor, and repeat. Do 16–18, then repeat to the other side.

Back of Thigh Toner Lie face down with your head resting on your hands, and your ankles crossed. Bend your knees and slowly raise your ankles off the floor, using the resistance of the top leg to make the exercise more difficult. Lower the ankles, and repeat. Do 16–18. Repeat with the other ankle on top.

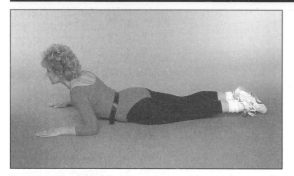

Tummy Stretch Lying face down with arms bent and legs together, slowly raise your head and shoulders off the floor, supporting yourself on your forearms and elbows. Feel the stretch down the front of your abdomen. Hold for 10 seconds.

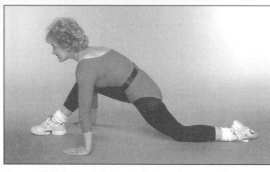

Upper Thigh Stretch Kneeling as shown, take your weight on to your front foot. Ease your hips forwards and feel the stretch in the front thigh of the back leg. Hold for 10 seconds, then relax, and repeat with the other leg.

Back of Thigh Stretch Resting on one knee, extend the other leg forwards and take your weight on to your hands placed at either side of your front leg. Ease your seat back towards your heel, but don't sit on it. Feel the stretch at the back of the front leg, and hold for 10 seconds. Relax, then change legs, and repeat.

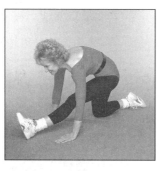

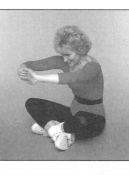

Upper Back Stretch Sitting with legs crossed, round your back and raise your arms in front to shoulder level to separate your shoulder blades. Hold for 10 seconds.

Waist Stretch Place one hand on the floor for support, and reach over to the side with the other arm. Hold for 10 seconds, then relax and repeat to the other side.

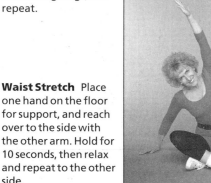

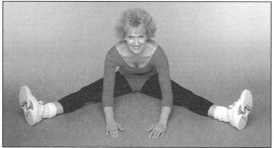

Advanced Inner Thigh Stretch Sitting with your legs wide apart and supporting your weight on your arms, ease your body forwards and feel the stretch in your inner thighs. Hold for 10 seconds.

POSITIVE THOUGHT FOR THE DAY

In these last two days I want to spend some time thinking about future goals and aspirations. As I start each new project there has to be some motivational factor to inspire me to give my very best. As each goal is achieved then another goal *has* to be created. What are *your* goals and what are *your* hopes and dreams? Go back to your original list of goals and keep reviewing that list and building upon it. Continue to record in your 'confidence book' all the good and positive things that you achieve and the compliments you receive. Look at your list of goals regularly to remind yourself of them as you try to redesign your life. Don't waste this life, it is too valuable and we can do so much good within it, not only for ourselves but for other people around us. Once you have committed your goals to paper you have in effect mapped out your future. If you are ready for success you will think a lot about them. You will be excited. You will plan how you are going to reach them and you will learn what you have to in order to do so. All of a sudden, you will find more energy, you will need less sleep, and you will be able to do more in your everyday life. You will find that the diet becomes easier to follow and that exercise becomes a regular part of your life. Remember, if you are to push forward towards your goals, each goal in itself must be regarded as a source of purpose, excitement and accomplishment, not confusion, disbelief and futility.

Be as physically active as you possibly can for the rest of the day and remember to maintain that good posture *all* the time. Get into the habit and you will look younger, taller and slimmer – all the time!

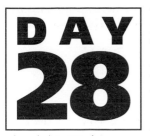

DAY 28

You've done it. You have actually done it! This is the most brilliant moment now that you have reached this last day. You must be *so* excited that you have almost completed this 28-day programme. You have had to gather every bit of willpower you could muster, and I hope you feel that all the effort has been worthwhile. You have just this one day to be very active and take extra care with your food so that you only eat the meals as suggested, with no extras. Don't forget that tomorrow is your final weighing and measuring day. Try on your skirt or trousers and see how much looser they are. Weigh and measure yourself and acknowledge the fantastic achievement you have made. If you need to lose more weight, then continue to select from any of the days' menus that you wish, and choose any of the daily exercise plans from this last week. Just continue until you reach what you consider to be your ideal weight. Don't aim to become too thin but realise at which weight you feel and look at your optimum. If you have reached your target weight, then follow the guidelines on maintenance eating detailed on page 180. Follow these simple rules and you will stay in great shape for the rest of your life.

Having achieved this magnificent first significant goal, look forward and upwards and keep going. Today's exercise plan is the most challenging yet but your body is now more than capable of completing it, and what you are able to achieve today is a far cry from what you could do 28 days ago. Give yourself a great big pat on the back and have a celebratory drink tonight.

MENU

BREAKFAST

4 fl oz (100 ml) orange juice; $1/_2$ oz (12.5 g) Bran Buds, 1 oz (25 g) All-Bran and 1 oz (25 g) sultanas with 4 fl oz (100 ml) milk (in addition to allowance)

or

1 slice melon chopped, 1 satsuma and 2 oz (50 g) canned or fresh pineapple cubed. Mix together and top with 4 tsp low-fat fromage frais

LUNCH

Ⓟ 1 cup of Batchelor's Slim a Soup; 2 pieces fresh fruit and 1 x 8 oz (200 g) pot Müllerlight yogurt

Ⓠ 2 oz (50 g) cold cooked beef or chicken, served with Coleslaw (page 179), jacket potato and salad

Ⓡ *Oriental Vegetable Soup* (page 159)
plus 1 slice wholemeal bread (no butter)

DINNER

STARTER
Wedge of melon

Ⓡ *Soufflé Potato and Ham Bake* (page 167)

Ⓠ 1 Bird's Eye Cod Steak in Parsley Sauce, served with unlimited vegetables

Ⓥ *Vegetable Casserole* (page 173)
served with additional vegetables if desired

DESSERT
Swiss Roll Meringue (page 179)

Extend alternate legs to the side, tapping the floor with your heels. Do 16.

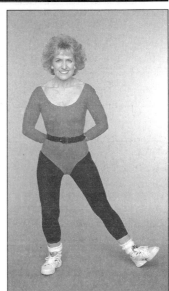

With feet a comfortable distance apart, raise one hip and at the same time raise the opposite shoulder. Repeat with the other hip and shoulder. Do 16 on alternate sides.

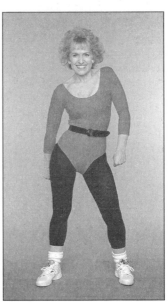

CONTINUED ▶

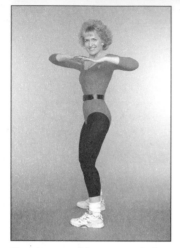 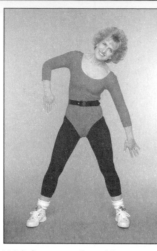 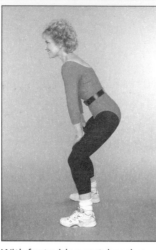 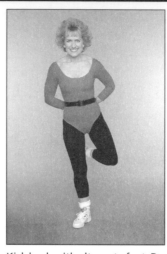 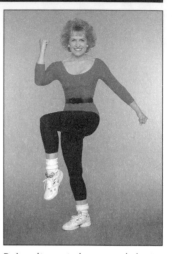

Keeping your hips square, twist your upper body from side to side. Do not jerk. Do 8 to each side.

With feet a comfortable distance apart, lean over to the side without twisting the hips. Repeat to the other side. Do 8 to each side.

With feet wide apart, bend your knees and go down into a squat, making sure the knees bend over the ankles. Come up again, and repeat. Do 8.

Kick back with alternate feet. Do 16.

Raise alternate knees and aim to touch with opposite elbow. Do 16.

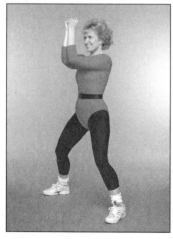 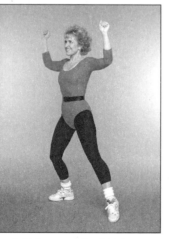 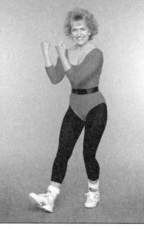 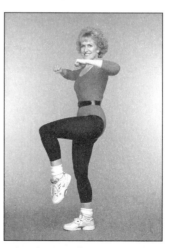

With feet wide apart, transfer your weight from one foot to the other, opening and closing your bent arms at shoulder level. Do 32.

Step from side to side and tap the opposite heel on the floor in front, flexing and straightening your arms as you step. Do 16.

Raise alternate knees, bringing both elbows back to draw your shoulder blades together with each raise. Do 32.

Bottom Streamliner
Holding on to the back of a chair, place your feet a comfortable distance apart, with your toes and knees facing slightly outwards. Bend your knees as if you were going to sit on a chair behind you, then straighten your knees and push your pelvis forwards, squeezing your buttocks together. Repeat 16–18 times.

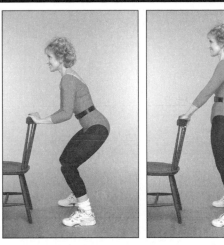
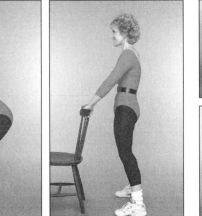

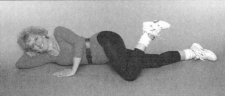
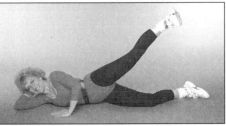

Outer Thigh Toner Lie on your side with both knees slightly bent. Dip the knee of the top leg on the floor in front and then, leading with the heel, extend and straighten it towards the corner of the room. Repeat this dipping and straightening movement 16–18 times, ensuring the hips remain square. Roll over, and repeat with the other leg.

Back of Thigh Toner Lie face down with your head resting on your hands, and your ankles crossed. Bend your knees and slowly raise your ankles off the floor, using the resistance of the top leg to make the exercise more difficult. Lower the ankles, and repeat. Do 16–18, then repeat with the other ankle on top.

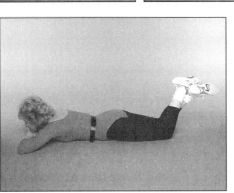

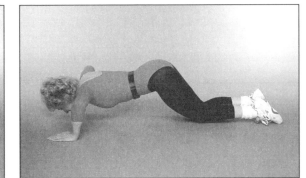

Chest Toner Position yourself on all fours and place your hands slightly wider than shoulder-width apart. Move your knees a little further away from your upper body to make the exercise more difficult. Keeping your chin in line with your fingers, lower your upper body towards the floor, then lift up again. Repeat as many times as possible without straining, proceeding at your own pace and according to your own strength. If necessary, take a rest, then continue.

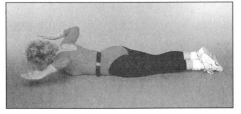

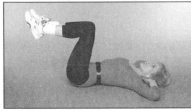

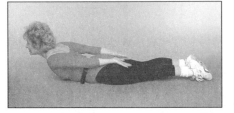

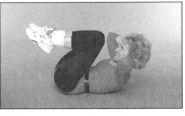

Upper Back Strengthener Lie face down with arms bent at shoulder level. Raise your arms, squeezing your shoulder blades together as much as possible. Lower your arms, and repeat. Do 16–18.

Back Strengthener Lying face down with legs together, place your hands on your seat. Slowly raise your chest and shoulders off the floor, using the muscles in your spine. Return to the floor, and repeat. Do 16–18.

Tummy Streamliner Lie on your back with knees bent and raised over your hips, and place your hands on either side of your head. *Pull your tummy in tightly* and lift your head and shoulders and, at the same time, bring your knees in towards your chest. Keep a distance between your chin and your chest. Return to the floor, and repeat. Do 16–18.

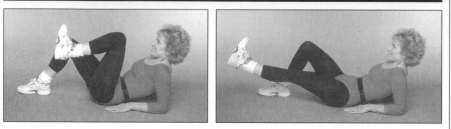

Front Thigh Toner Supporting yourself on your arms, bend both knees. Bring one knee in towards your chest and then extend the leg straight out in front. Keep your tummy tight to support your back. Bring the leg towards your chest again, and repeat. Do 16–18, then repeat with the other leg.

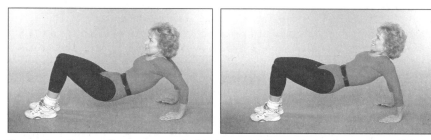

Upper Arm Toner Place your arms behind you with fingers facing forwards, and lift your hips off the floor so that your weight is supported by your feet and your hands. Now, straighten your arms to raise your hips further and try to straighten your body as much as possible. Lower your hips without returning completely to the floor. Continue to raise and lower your body, and repeat as many times as possible

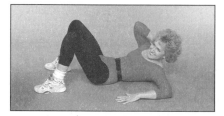

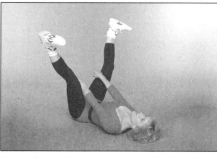

Waist Toner Lying on your back with knees bent, place one hand behind your neck and have the other arm on the floor for support. Raise your head and shoulder and bring your elbow towards the opposite knee, taking care not to roll your hips. Return to the floor, and repeat. Do 16–18, then repeat to the other side.

Inner Thigh Toner Lie on your back with your feet raised above your hips, legs apart, and hands on the inside of your thighs. Use your hands for resistance as you aim to bring your legs together. Do 16.

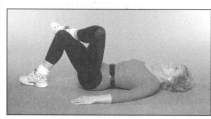

Back of Thigh Stretch Lying on your back with knees bent, take hold of one leg and raise it, straightening it as far as is comfortable. Ease the leg towards you with your hands and hold for 10–15 seconds. Relax, and repeat with the other leg.

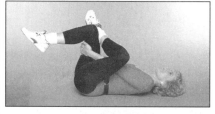

Outer Thigh Stretch Still lying on your back, bend one knee and place the other leg in front of it. Place one hand through the middle of your legs and the other hand round the outside of the bottom leg. Slowly ease your legs towards your chest, and feel the stretch in the outer thigh of the top leg. Hold for 10 seconds, then relax and change legs to repeat on the other side.

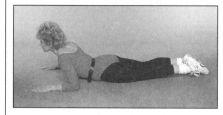

Tummy Stretch Lie face down and place your arms to the sides with elbows bent. Slowly raise your head and shoulders off the floor, supporting yourself on your forearms and elbows, and feel the stretch down the front of your abdomen. Hold for 10 seconds.

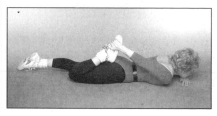

Front Thigh Stretch Resting your head on one hand, bend the opposite leg and use your hand to ease it towards your seat. Hold for 10 seconds then release, and repeat with the other leg.

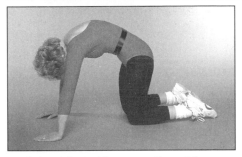

Back Stretch Position yourself on all fours and arch the spine as much as possible, pulling your tummy towards your spine. Hold for 10 seconds.

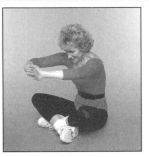

Upper Back Stretch Sitting with legs crossed, round your back and raise your arms in front to shoulder level to separate your shoulder blades. Hold for 10 seconds.

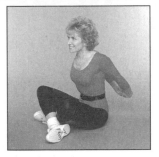

Chest Stretch Raise your arms and clasp your hands behind your back to stretch the muscles across your chest. Hold for 10 seconds.

Advanced Inner Thigh Stretch Sitting with your legs wide apart and supporting your weight on your arms, ease your body forwards and feel the stretch in your inner thighs. Hold for 10 seconds.

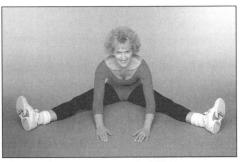

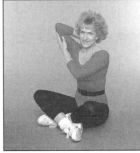

Back of Upper Arm Stretch Raise one elbow and ease your hand down your back. Use the other arm to ease it further. Hold for 10 seconds. Repeat with the other arm.

Waist and Outer Thigh Stretch Sit up straight with one leg extended and the other leg placed across it. Slowly twist your body away from the bent knee, using the opposite elbow to ease the bent knee further across. Hold for 10 seconds, then change legs and repeat to the other side.

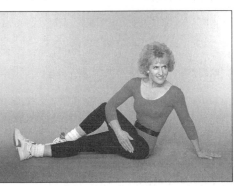

POSITIVE THOUGHT FOR THE DAY

On this final day I feel it is appropriate to sum up the thoughts and ideas we have covered over the last few weeks. I owe a great deal to the successful people from whom I have learnt so much. Here are my basic guidelines to achieving *your* goals. Follow them and, honestly, you can't fail:

1 Goals must be believable.
2 Goals must be clearly defined and understood.
3 You must want your goals badly enough.
4 Goals must be put down in writing.
5 You should stipulate a date to indicate the time by which you hope to achieve each goal. These dates can be altered, but do give your goals a timescale.
6 Keep looking back at your goal list. Constantly remind yourself of them. Tick off those that have been achieved and remind yourself of those achievements.
7 Set yourself different goals for different timescales, for instance, a goal for next week, a goal for one month's time, three months' time, a year or three years' time and, of course, your ultimate goal.
8 Remember to *live* for today. Don't worry about tomorrow, but don't put off till tomorrow what you can do today.
9 Make keeping trim and fit one of your goals. Achieve this, and your confidence will rocket sky high and your other goals will be so much easier to accomplish. Don't ever underestimate the value of believing in yourself and liking yourself. Start behaving like the person you want to be.
10 Learn to laugh and smile and enjoy each day, living life to the full and never wasting a moment by being negative.

We need to *look* for a wonderful life. If it isn't wonderful for you yet, it soon will be. So go for it!

Recipes

STARTERS

Cheesy Pears
(Serves 1)

1 ripe pear
lemon juice
2 oz (50 g) low-fat cottage cheese
shredded lettuce

Peel, halve lengthways and core the pear. Brush with lemon juice to prevent discoloration. Fill the cavities with the cottage cheese, and serve on a bed of shredded lettuce.

Chicken Liver Pâté with Brandy
(Serves 6)

8 oz (200 g) frozen chicken livers,
defrosted and rinsed
4 oz (100 g) mushrooms, sliced
1 onion, peeled and chopped
1 clove garlic, peeled
4 slices lean back bacon, chopped
2 tsp tomato purée
2 pinches mixed herbs
3 tbsp water
salt and black pepper to taste
1 tbsp brandy
salad and lemon wedges to garnish

For the melba toast
6 thin slices bread

Wash the chicken livers in cold water and drain well. Place all the ingredients, except the brandy, into a non-metallic dish and microwave on *full* power for 10 minutes and then *low* power for 5 minutes, stirring occasionally.

Leave to stand for 10 minutes, then add the brandy. Place in a food processor and blend until the mixture is either slightly rough or smooth, according to preference.

Turn out into an oblong container (a margarine tub is ideal) and chill thoroughly in the fridge.

To make melba toast, toast the bread in a toaster. As soon as it pops up, cut the slice in half horizontally using a sharp knife. Arrange on a grill tray untoasted side up, and brown.

Cut the pâté into slices and garnish with salad and lemon wedges. Serve with 1 slice melba toast per person.

Crispy Garlic Mushrooms
(Serves 3)

6 large mushrooms
2–3 cloves garlic, peeled and crushed
5 oz (125 g) low-fat natural yogurt
4 oz (100 g) fresh breadcrumbs
salt and black pepper to taste

Wipe the mushrooms and remove the stalks. Mix the garlic with the yogurt.

Dip each mushroom into the yogurt using a pastry brush to cover them fully, then dip into the breadcrumbs.

Place on a non-stick baking tray and bake in a preheated oven at 200°C, 400°F, or Gas Mark 6 for 10–15 minutes.

Add salt and pepper to the remaining yogurt and serve with the mushrooms.

Serve with tomato and cucumber salad.

Note: The yogurt sauce mix is even better if made the previous day and chilled in the refrigerator overnight. Keep covered.

French Tomatoes
(Serves 4)

8 tomatoes
6 oz (150 g) low-fat cottage cheese
small bunch of fresh chives or spring onion tops or parsley, finely chopped
salt and black pepper to taste
Oil-free Vinaigrette Dressing (page 179)
watercress to garnish

Scald and skin the tomatoes by placing them in a bowl, pouring boiling water over them and counting to fifteen before pouring off the hot water and replacing it with cold. The skin then comes off easily.

Cut a slice from the non-stalk end of each tomato and reserve the slices. Hold a tomato in the palm of your hand and remove the seeds with the handle of a teaspoon, then remove the core with the bowl of the spoon. Repeat with the remaining tomatoes. Drain the hollowed-out tomatoes and season lightly inside each one with salt.

Soften the cheese with a fork. When soft, add most of the finely chopped chives, spring onion tops or parsley and season well. Fill the tomatoes with the cheese mixture, using a small teaspoon, until the mixture is above the rim of each tomato. Replace their top slices on the slant and arrange the tomatoes in a serving dish.

Spoon most of the dressing over the tomatoes, reserving some to add just before serving. Chill the tomatoes for up to 2 hours. Before serving, garnish with watercress and sprinkle the remaining chives and dressing over the tomatoes.

Garlic and Mint Yogurt Dip with Crudités

(Serves 4)

5 oz (125 g) low-fat natural yogurt
1 clove garlic, peeled and finely chopped
2 sprigs fresh mint, chopped
4 oz (100 g) low-fat cottage cheese

Crudités
Sticks and sprigs of raw cucumber,
carrots, celery, green and
red peppers and cauliflower

Mix the yogurt, garlic, mint and cottage cheese together. Serve in a small dish, accompanied by crudités.

Grilled Grapefruit

(Serves 2)

1 grapefruit
2 tbsp sweet sherry
2 tsp brown sugar

Cut the grapefruit in half. Using a grapefruit knife, remove the core and membranes between segments. Pour the sherry over the flesh, and sprinkle brown sugar over. Place in a heatproof dish, and then place under a hot grill until the sugar is glazed.

Serve hot.

Orange and Grapefruit Cocktail

(Serves 2)

1 large orange
1 grapefruit

Remove all peel and pith from both fruits. Work the segments from the core with a sharp knife and arrange in two dishes. Squeeze as much juice as possible on to the fruit from the peel and core.

Serve chilled.

Melon and Prawn Salad

(Serves 2)

1 melon
4 oz (100 g) prawns, shelled

Halve the melon and remove the seeds. Scoop out the flesh with a ball-scoop. Mix the melon balls carefully with the shelled prawns, and replace in the empty melon shells.

Serve chilled.

Marinated Haddock

(Serves 4)

12 oz (300 g) uncooked smoked haddock
1 medium onion, peeled and cut into rings
1–2 small carrots, trimmed and scraped,
cut into julienne sticks
1 tsp coriander seeds
2 bay leaves
2 lemons, plus extra lemon juice if necessary
2 tbsp white wine vinegar or cider vinegar
1 tsp caster sugar
few lettuce leaves
4 slices lemon and 4 sprigs fresh parsley
or chervil to garnish

Skin the haddock and remove any bones. Cut the fish into finger-sized strips (2$\frac{1}{2}$ x $\frac{1}{2}$ in/5 x 1 cm) and place in a shallow dish. Spread the onion, carrots and coriander seeds over the fish, and tuck the bay leaves under it.

Grate the zest from 1 lemon and squeeze the juice from both. Measure the juice and, if necessary, make up to 4 fl oz (100 ml) with extra juice. Mix the juice with the grated zest and vinegar, and pour over the fish. Sprinkle the caster sugar over the top. Cover and refrigerate for 8 hours or overnight.

To serve, arrange a few lettuce leaves on individual dishes. Remove the bay leaves and place a quarter of the fish and vegetables in the centre of each dish. Pour over a little of the marinade. Garnish each dish, if you wish, with a twist of lemon and a sprig of parsley or chervil. Refrigerate until required.

Mussels in White Wine

(Serves 4)

4$\frac{1}{2}$ lb (2 kg) mussels
1 small onion, peeled and finely chopped
1 clove garlic, peeled and crushed, or $\frac{1}{2}$ tsp garlic
paste (optional)
few parsley stalks
1 sprig thyme
$\frac{1}{4}$ pint/5 fl oz (125 ml) dry white wine,
or dry cider if preferred
black pepper to taste
1–2 tbsp chopped fresh parsley to garnish

Wash the mussels well in several changes of water until they are free of sand and grit. Discard any which are broken or which remain open after being plunged into cold water or given a sharp tap. With a small knife, scrape the barnacles off the shells and remove the beards (the black threads hanging from the mussels).

Place the onion and garlic in a large pan with the parsley stalks, thyme and dry white wine (or cider). Cover and simmer gently for about 5 minutes until the onion is nearly tender.

Add the mussels, season with black pepper, cover and cook for a further 5–7 minutes over a good heat, shaking the pan occasionally until all the mussels are open. If the odd mussel remains closed, discard it.

Pile the mussels into a large serving bowl or individual dishes. Pour the cooking liquor over, discarding the last few spoonfuls as these may contain grit. Sprinkle the mussels with chopped fresh parsley and serve immediately.

Carrot and Tarragon Soup

(Serves 4–6)

1$\frac{1}{2}$ pints/30 fl oz (750 ml) chicken stock
made with 1 stock cube
12 oz (300 g) carrots, trimmed, scraped and grated
8 oz (200 g) potatoes, peeled and grated
1 onion, peeled and finely chopped or grated
1 tbsp tarragon
salt and black pepper to taste
5 oz (125 g) low-fat natural yogurt

Place all the ingredients, except for the yogurt, in a large saucepan. Bring to the boil and simmer for about 1 hour until cooked or tender. Remove from the heat and liquidise in a blender or food processor until smooth.

Place in a warm serving dish, and stir in the yogurt just before serving.

Chicken and Sweetcorn Soup
(Serves 4)

6 oz (150 g) cooked chicken
1 x 12 oz (300 g) can 'light' sweetcorn, drained
1 x 12 oz (300 g) can 'creamed' sweetcorn, drained
2 pints (1 litre) chicken stock or 2 chicken stock
cubes in 2 pints (1 litre) water
$^1/_2$ tsp crushed chilli seeds
or 1 tsp chilli sauce (optional)
salt and black pepper to taste
2 egg whites
1 level tbsp cornflour
chopped chives to garnish

Cut the chicken into small pieces. Place the chicken, the contents of both cans of sweetcorn and the stock in a large saucepan. Gently bring to the boil, reduce the heat and simmer for 15 minutes.

Add the chilli and seasoning.

Gradually add the egg whites, stirring briskly, in order to create 'strands'. Mix the cornflour with a little water, then slowly blend into the soup mixture, stirring continuously.

Garnish with a few chopped chives before serving.

Chunky Vegetable Soup
(Serves 6)

2 small carrots, thinly sliced
2 leeks, thinly sliced
1–2 parsnips, diced into $^1/_4$ inch (5 mm) cubes
1–2 sticks celery, thinly sliced
1 medium onion, thinly sliced
$^1/_4$–$^1/_2$ medium swede, diced into $^1/_4$ inch (5 mm) cubes
few dark green cabbage leaves, chopped
1 x 16 oz (400 g) can chopped tomatoes
1 clove garlic, peeled and chopped or crushed
1 bay leaf
2 level tsp salt
2–3 pints (1–2 litres) vegetable stock
2 oz (50 g) small pasta shapes (optional)
1 level tsp dried oregano (optional)
black pepper to taste

Place all the vegetables together with the chopped tomatoes in a very large pan. Add the garlic, bay leaf, salt and vegetable stock.

Bring to the boil and simmer for 1–1$^1/_2$ hours, until the vegetables are tender.

To add an Italian touch, add the pasta shapes and dried oregano 20 minutes before the end of the cooking time.

Remove the bay leaf and discard. Season to taste.

If a thick soup is preferred place half the vegetables in a liquidiser, purée, then stir back into the remaining vegetables.

Cream of Leek and Potato Soup
(Serves 6)

2 large potatoes, scrubbed and diced (do not peel)
2 large leeks, washed and sliced
(use as many of the dark leaves as possible)
1 large onion, peeled and finely chopped
2 cloves garlic, crushed (optional)
1 pint/20 fl oz (500 ml) skimmed or semi-skimmed
milk (in addition to allowance)
1 sachet bouquet garni
1 chicken stock cube, dissolved in a little hot water
black pepper to taste
2 tsp cornflour
1 level tsp salt
chopped fresh parsley to garnish

Place all the vegetables (including the garlic if used) in a large pan. Add the milk, bouquet garni, stock cube and pepper.

Stir well, bring to the boil and simmer gently for $^3/_4$ hour. Remove the bouquet garni and discard.

Mix the cornflour with a little water and blend carefully into the soup, stirring continuously. Place in a food processor or blender and liquidise until smooth, adding more water if the soup is too thick. Season to taste.

Garnish with chopped parsley before serving.

Creamy Vegetable Soup
(Serves 4)

1$^1/_4$ lb (500 g) potatoes, peeled and diced
8 oz (200 g) carrots, trimmed, scraped and sliced
2 leeks, finely chopped
2$^1/_2$ pints (1.5 litres) vegetable stock
salt and black pepper to taste
2 oz (50 g) skimmed milk powder
(in addition to allowance)
1 oz (25 g) cornflour
fresh chopped parsley to garnish

Place all the vegetables in a saucepan with the stock. Season, cover and simmer for 20–30 minutes.

Blend the skimmed milk powder and cornflour with a little cold water and stir into the soup. Bring to the boil and simmer for 5 minutes, stirring continuously.

Garnish with chopped parsley before serving.

Haricot Bean and Vegetable Soup
(Serves 4–6)

4 oz (100 g) haricot beans
4 oz (100 g) orange split peas
2 pints (1 litre) vegetable stock
(saved from vegetables cooked previously
or made up with a vegetable stock cube)
4 oz (100 g) country soup mixture
1 chicken stock cube
2 carrots, trimmed, scraped and diced
1 parsnip, peeled and diced
1 medium onion, peeled and chopped
1 stick celery, sliced
1 clove garlic, peeled and crushed
salt and black pepper to taste
chopped fresh parsley to garnish

Soak the haricot beans and orange split peas overnight in the vegetable stock.

Place the beans and peas and country soup mixture into a large saucepan and add the remaining ingredients. Bring to the boil, remove any sediment and simmer for about 2 hours, adding more water if required.

Season to taste. Pour into a serving dish and garnish with chopped parsley. Ideally, leave to stand overnight before serving.

Oriental Vegetable Soup
(Serves 4)

1 small red pepper, deseeded anc chopped
1 small yellow pepper, deseeded and chopped
1 medium leek, chopped
1 clove garlic, peeled and crushed
1 tsp fresh ginger, peeled and grated
1 stick celery, sliced
1 medium carrot, trimmed, scraped
and cut into rings
4 oz (100 g) Savoy cabbage, shredded
10 oz (250 g) potatoes, peeled and cut into strips
$1^{3}/_{4}$ pints (1 litre) vegetable stock
salt and black pepper to taste
2 oz (50 g) bean sprouts
1 tsp soy sauce

Place all the vegetables except the bean sprouts in a large non-stock saucepan and dry-fry until they begin to soften.

Add the stock, bring to the boil and season well. Reduce the heat, cover and simmer for 10–15 minutes until the potatoes are just cooked.

Add the bean sprouts and cook for 5 minutes. Readjust the seasoning and stir in the soy sauce. Serve immediately.

Potato and Watercress Soup
(Serves 4)

1 onion, peeled and chopped
2 bunches watercress, chopped
1 lb (400 g) potatoes, peeled and diced
1 pint/20 fl oz (500 ml) chicken stock
salt and black pepper to taste
$1/_{4}$ pint/5 fl oz (125 ml) semi-skimmed
or skimmed milk (in addition to allowance)

Dry-fry the onion in a non-stick frying pan until soft. Add the watercress and potatoes and fry for a further minute. Pour in the stock. Season, bring to the boil and simmer for 30 minutes.

Remove from the heat, then sieve or liquidise and return to the saucepan. Add the milk. Reheat, but do not boil.

Tomato and Orange Soup
(Serves 4)

1 large onion, peeled and grated
1 large carrot, trimmed, scraped and grated
1 x 14 oz (350 g) can chopped tomatoes
8 oz (200 g) potatoes, peeled and thinly sliced
1 tsp mixed herbs
$1/_{2}$ tsp demerara sugar
zest and juice of 1 orange
1 pint/20 fl oz (500 ml) chicken stock
salt and black pepper to taste
5 oz (125 g) low-fat natural yogurt
parsley sprigs to garnish

In a non-stick saucepan gently dry-fry the onion for 5 minutes then add the grated carrot and cook for 2 more minutes.

Add all the other ingredients except the yogurt, and simmer gently for 30 minutes.

Liquidise the soup in a blender, or pass through a sieve. Add the yogurt, adjust the seasoning and reheat, but do not boil. Garnish with parsley sprigs, and serve.

Watercress Soup
(Serves 4)

1 pint/20 fl oz (500 ml) chicken stock made using 2
stock cubes
$1/_{2}$ bunch watercress
1 shallot, peeled
salt and black pepper to taste
2 dashes Worcester sauce (optional)
1 level tbsp cornflour, mixed to a paste with water

Wash the watercress very thoroughly in cold water. Place all the ingredients, except the cornflour, in a blender and blend for 30 seconds.

Remove from the blender and heat in a saucepan or microwave to boiling point. Mix in the cornflour and bring back to the boil. Serve immediately.

For a stronger flavour use a whole bunch of watercress.

LUNCHES

American Turkey Burgers
(Serves 4)

3 level tbsp dry sage and onion stuffing mix
3 tbsp boiling water
12 oz (300 g) fresh turkey mince
1 egg white
1/2 medium onion, peeled and chopped
salt and black pepper to taste

Stir the stuffing mix into the water in a large bowl and leave to stand for 1 minute.

Add the turkey, egg white and onion, and season to taste.

Mix well, then, using your hands, divide the mixture into 8 balls and press into burger shapes (or use a burger press). Place on a plate and leave to chill in the refrigerator for at least 15 minutes.

Grill under a medium heat, turning frequently, for about 20 minutes or until golden brown. Ensure the burgers are cooked throughout.

Serve in a burger bun (1 x 2 oz/50 g bun per person) with unlimited salad, tomato and relish.

Beefburger in Bun
(Serves 4)

1 lb (400 g) minced beef
1 large onion, peeled and finely chopped
3 tbsp breadcrumbs
4 tbsp milk (in addition to allowance)
4 burger buns
4 tomato slices
tomato ketchup

Mix the minced beef, chopped onion, breadcrumbs and milk in a large bowl. Leave to stand for 10 minutes.

Divide the mixture into 4 balls and press into burger shapes.

Cook under a preheated hot grill for 5 minutes each side.

Place each burger in a bun with a slice of tomato and tomato ketchup.

Chinese Apple Salad
(Serves 1)

1 red apple, thinly sliced
1 green apple, thinly sliced
1 tbsp lemon juice
6 oz (150 g) fresh bean sprouts
few radishes, sliced
2 sticks celery, sliced
1 bunch spring onions, sliced
curly lettuce to decorate

Sweet and Sour Dressing
1 1/2 tbsp lemon juice
1 level tbsp clear honey
few drops soy sauce

In a salad bowl, mix the apples and lemon juice thoroughly, then add the bean sprouts, radishes, celery and spring onions.

Decorate the edge of the bowl with curly lettuce.

Mix together the dressing ingredients and pour over the salad. Toss well and serve immediately.

Fruit and Chicken Salad
(Serves 1)

Unlimited amounts of shredded lettuce, chopped cucumber, peppers and any other green salad items
1 apple, peeled, cored and sliced
1 pear, peeled, cored and sliced
1 orange, peeled and segmented
1 kiwi fruit, peeled and sliced
2 oz (50 g) cooked chicken breast, chopped
2 tbsp low-fat natural yogurt
1 tbsp wine vinegar
1 clove garlic, peeled and crushed
salt and black pepper to taste

Place the lettuce and green salad on to a large dinner plate.

Lay the slices of fruit in a circle on top of the salad vegetables and place the chopped chicken in the centre.

To make the dressing mix the yogurt with the wine vinegar and garlic, and season to taste. Pour the dressing over the salad, and serve.

Jacket Potato with Curried Chicken and Yogurt Topping
(Serves 1)

3 oz (75 g) low-fat natural yogurt
1 tsp curry powder
2 oz (50 g) cooked chicken breast, cut into cubes
1 medium sized (8 oz/200 g) jacket potato, cooked

Mix the yogurt and curry powder together and stir in the cubes of cooked chicken. Cut open the cooked jacket potato and top with curried chicken mixture. Serve with unlimited green salad items.

Jacket Potato with Onion Mushrooms
(Serves 2)

1 medium onion, peeled and chopped
1/2 vegetable stock cube dissolved in 2 tbsp boiling water
12 oz (300 g) closed cup mushrooms, sliced
pepper to taste
2 x 8 oz (200 g) jacket potatoes, cooked
chopped parsley to garnish

Place the chopped onion and stock in a frying pan, cover and simmer gently until the onion softens.

Add the mushrooms and seasoning and cook, uncovered, for approximately 15 minutes or until the juice has reduced slightly.

Pile into the cooked jacket potatoes, and sprinkle with chopped parsley.

Serve with unlimited salad items.

DINNERS

MEAT AND POULTRY

Beef Bourguignon
(Serves 4)

16 oz (400 g) stewing beef
2 medium onions, peeled and sliced
2 carrots, trimmed, scraped and sliced
4 oz (100 g) button mushrooms
1 x 1^1/$_2$ oz (40 g) sachet Colman's Beef Bourguignon
Casserole Mix

Place the beef, onions, carrots and mushrooms into an ovenproof dish.

Mix the contents of the casserole mix sachet with ^{3}/$_4$ pint/15 fl oz (475 ml) water and stir into the dish. Cover and cook in a preheated oven at 180°C, 350°C, or Gas Mark 4 for about 1^1/$_2$ hours or until the beef is tender.

Serve with unlimited vegetables and potatoes.

Beef Casserole
(Serves 4)

16 oz (400 g) stewing beef
2 medium onions, peeled and sliced
2 large carrots, trimmed, scraped and sliced
1 x 1^1/$_2$ oz (40 g) sachet Colman's Traditional Beef
Casserole Mix

Place the beef into an ovenproof dish. Add the onions and carrots.

Mix the contents of the casserole mix sachet with ^{3}/$_4$ pint/15 fl oz (475 ml) water and stir into the dish. Cover and cook in a preheated oven at 180°C, 350°F, or Gas Mark 4 for 1^3/$_4$ hours or until the beef is tender.

Serve with unlimited vegetables and potatoes.

Spaghetti Bolognese
(Serves 4)

16 oz (400 g) lean minced beef
1 medium onion, peeled and finely chopped
2 cloves garlic, peeled and crushed
1 x 14^1/$_2$ oz (360 g) jar bolognese sauce
(e.g. Dolmio, Ragu or Homepride)

Dry-fry the mince in a non-stick frying pan. Remove from the pan, drain well and put to one side. Discard any fat from the pan, then add the onion and dry-fry until brown. Return the mince to the pan, add the garlic and heat through. Add the bolognese sauce and simmer for 10 minutes.

Serve with spaghetti (2 oz/50 g [dry weight] per person).

Lamb Kebabs with Onion Sauce
(Serves 4)

1 onion, peeled
^{1}/$_2$ pint/10 fl oz (250 ml) semi-skimmed
or skimmed milk (in addition to allowance)
1 lb (400 g) lean lamb, cubed
1 green pepper, deseeded and cut into 1 inch
(2.5 cm) pieces
8 button mushrooms
8 cherry tomatoes or 4 tomatoes, halved
1 tbsp cornflour
salt and black pepper to taste

Cut the onion into 8 pieces and put into a small saucepan. Reserve 2 tablespoons of the milk, and add the rest to the pan. Bring to the boil. Simmer gently for about 15 minutes until the onion is soft.

Prepare the kebabs by threading the meat and vegetables on to skewers. Cook under a preheated grill for 10–15 minutes, turning frequently.

To complete the onion sauce, blend the cornflour with the reserved milk. Add to the cooked onion and milk and bring to the boil, stirring continuously. Season. Serve with the kebabs.

Serve with boiled brown rice (2 oz/50 g [dry weight] per person).

Campfire Kidneys
(Serves 4)

1 lb (400 g) new potatoes, well scrubbed and halved
8 lamb kidneys, skinned, cored and halved
1 oz (25 g) plain flour, seasoned
1 medium onion, peeled and roughly chopped
1 clove garlic, peeled and crushed
1 x 14 oz (350 g) can tomatoes
1 tbsp tomato purée
1 tbsp sherry
salt and black pepper to taste
1 x 7 oz (175 g) can sweetcorn, drained
4 oz (100 g) button mushrooms

Place the potatoes into just enough boiling water to cover, and cook gently until just tender. Drain and set aside.

Toss the kidneys in a little of the seasoned flour until well coated.

Dry-fry the onion and garlic in a non-stick frying pan until soft. Add 2 tablespoons of the tomato juice from the canned tomatoes.

Add the kidneys and cook for a further 5 minutes.

Add the remaining flour together with the tomatoes, tomato purée and sherry, and season well. Simmer for 10 minutes.

Add the sweetcorn, mushrooms and potatoes and simmer for a further 15 minutes until the kidneys are tender.

Serve with unlimited fresh green vegetables.

Chinese Menu 1

Beef in Black Bean Sauce
Sweet and Sour Pork
Chicken in Spicy Tomato Sauce
(Serves 4)

4 oz (100 g) lean beef steak
4 oz (100 g) lean pork
8 oz (200 g) chicken breast
2 medium onions, peeled and chopped
1 green pepper, deseeded and chopped
1 x 8 oz (200 g) can water chestnuts
3 cloves garlic, peeled and crushed
1 sachet Blue Dragon Canton Black Bean Sauce
1 sachet Blue Dragon Sweet and Sour Sauce
1 sachet Blue Dragon Szechuan Spicy Tomato Sauce
8 oz (200 g) bean sprouts
8 oz (200 g) [dry weight] rice

Chop the beef, pork and chicken into bite-size pieces and dry-fry in three separate non-stick pans.

When the meat has changed colour add to each pan equal quantities of the chopped onion. Add the chopped pepper to the pork and beef dishes, and the water chestnuts to the chicken and pork dishes. Add a clove of garlic to each pan, then add the contents of each sachet of sauce to its respective pan.

Continue to cook for a further 5 minutes, and in the last minute before serving add the bean sprouts to the pork and beef dishes.

Meanwhile boil the rice according to the instructions on the packet. When cooked, drain through a colander.

Serve the meat in three individual dishes with the boiled rice served separately.

Chinese Menu 2

Singapore Beef Curry
Chicken in Orange and Green Ginger Sauce
Prawns in Yellow Bean Sauce
(Serves 4)

6 oz (150 g) lean beef, cut into cubes
8 oz (200 g) chicken breast,
skinned and chopped into cubes
6 oz (150 g) prawns, peeled and washed
1 large green pepper, cored, deseeded
and thinly sliced
1 large Spanish onion, peeled and chopped
1 sachet Blue Dragon Orange
and Green Ginger Sauce
1 x 8 oz (200 g) can bamboo shoots
1 sachet Blue Dragon Singapore Curry Sauce
1 sachet Blue Dragon Yellow Bean Sauce

Dry-fry the beef, chicken and prawns in three separate non-stick pans, seasoning well as you cook.

Add the slices of thin strips of green pepper and a third of the chopped Spanish onion to the chopped chicken dish. When the chicken has changed colour add the orange and green ginger sauce and simmer for a further 10 minutes.

Meanwhile add a third of the chopped Spanish onion to the beef, and season well. When the beef has changed colour add half the can of bamboo shoots and the Singapore curry sauce, and simmer for a further 10 minutes.

To the prawns in the third pan add the remaining bamboo shoots and chopped onion. Add the yellow bean sauce and simmer gently for 5 minutes.

When cooked, place each in a separate serving dish and serve with boiled brown rice (2 oz/50 g [dry weight] per person).

Apricot-glazed Chicken
(Serves 8)

1 x 13$\frac{1}{2}$ oz (336 g) jar apricot preserve
1 tbsp mayonnaise
1 tbsp tomato ketchup
$\frac{1}{4}$ tsp dry mustard
8 chicken breasts, boned and skinned
1 tbsp low-fat margarine
4 oz (100 g) onions, peeled and finely chopped
4 oz (100 g) celery, finely chopped
2 oz (50 g) mushrooms, sliced
$\frac{1}{4}$ pint/5 fl oz (125 ml) chicken stock
5 oz (125 g) Bran Buds cereal
8 oz (200 g) water chestnuts, chopped
$\frac{1}{2}$ tsp salt
$\frac{1}{4}$ tsp black pepper
$\frac{1}{4}$ tsp sage

Combine the preserve, mayonnaise, ketchup and dry mustard. Set aside.

Place each chicken breast between waxed paper. Pound the flesh to $\frac{1}{8}$ inch (0.3 cm) thickness, taking care not to tear it. Set aside.

Melt the margarine in a medium-sized frying pan. Add the onions and celery. Stirring frequently, cook over a medium heat until crisp-tender. Stir in the mushrooms and cook for a further 3–4 minutes.

Combine the chicken stock with the Bran Buds cereal and leave to stand for about 1 minute or until the cereal has absorbed the stock.

Mix the vegetables, water chestnuts, salt, pepper and sage into the cereal mixture and use to stuff each chicken breast. Roll each breast up, folding the ends and place seam-side down in a 12 x 8 inch (80 x 30 cm) shallow baking dish. Spoon the sauce over the chicken rolls.

Bake uncovered in a preheated oven at 180°C, 350°F, or Gas Mark 4 for about 45 minutes or until the chicken is tender.

Serve with unlimited vegetables and potatoes.

Basil, Chilli and Chicken Stir-fry

(Serves 4)

$1\frac{1}{2}$ lb (600 g) chicken breast
2 red peppers, deseeded and thinly sliced
$\frac{1}{2}$ can bamboo shoots, drained and thinly sliced
1 x 6 oz (155 g) jar Sharwood's Stir-fry Basil
and Chilli Sauce

Chop the chicken and dry-fry in a non-stick frying pan for 3 minutes. Add the red peppers, bamboo shoots and the basil and chilli sauce. Stir-fry for 3 further minutes.

Serve with boiled brown rice (2 oz/50 g [dry weight] per person).

Chicken Chasseur

(Serves 4)

4 chicken portions or 1 lb (400 g) cubed chicken
1 x 15 oz (375 g) can Homepride Chicken
Chasseur Sauce

Place the chicken in an ovenproof casserole dish. Pour the sauce over and stir in. Cover and cook in a pre-heated oven at 160°C, 325°F, or Gas Mark 3 for approximately $1\frac{1}{2}$ hours or until the meat is tender. Stir gently once or twice during cooking.

Alternatively, place in a microwave casserole dish, pour the sauce over and stir in. Cook on *full* power for 14–18 minutes according to the power rating of your microwave. Stir carefully halfway through the cooking time. Leave to stand for 2 minutes, stir well and serve.

Serve with unlimited vegetables and potatoes.

Chicken Chop Suey

(Serves 4)

$1\frac{1}{2}$ lb (600 g) chicken breast
1 medium carrot, trimmed, scraped and coarsely
grated
1 x $1\frac{1}{2}$ oz (32 g) sachet Schwartz World Cuisine
Mix for Chop Suey
8 oz (200 g) fresh bean sprouts
1 bunch spring onions
1 tsp dark soy sauce

Chop the chicken and place together with the carrot in a non-stick frying pan. Dry-fry until almost cooked.

Mix the contents of the chop suey mix sachet in – pint/10 fl oz (250 ml) water and stir into the pan. Add the bean sprouts, spring onions and soy sauce. Bring to the boil, then simmer uncovered for 2 minutes or until the meat is tender.

Serve with boiled brown rice (2 oz/50 g [dry weight] per person).

Chicken Dhansak

(Serves 2)

1 onion, peeled and chopped
2 cloves garlic, peeled and crushed
$\frac{1}{2}$ tsp turmeric
1 tbsp curry powder
1 tbsp tomato purée
$\frac{1}{4}$ pint/5 fl oz (125 ml) chicken stock
1 x 16 oz (400 g) can lentil soup
8 oz (200 g) cooked chicken chopped into bite-size
pieces

For the onion salad
1 small onion, peeled and sliced thinly into rings
1 tomato, chopped
$\frac{1}{2}$ tsp mint sauce

Dry-fry the onion and garlic in a pan over a medium heat until soft. Add the turmeric, curry powder and tomato purée. Mix well and add the stock and soup. Bring to the boil and simmer for 10 minutes, stirring occasionally.

Add the cooked chicken and simmer for a further 5 minutes or until the chicken is warmed through.

Mix the salad ingredients together.

Serve the chicken mixture on a bed of boiled brown rice (2 oz/50 g [dry weight] per person) with the onion salad.

Note: This recipe can be adapted for vegetarians substituting a selection of vegetables and chickpeas for the chicken.

Chicken with Herby Lemon Sauce

(Serves 4–6)

1 medium-sized roasting chicken
1 lemon, cut into slices
grated zest and juice of 1 lemon
few sprigs of fresh thyme and fresh parsley, chopped
2 tsp cornflour
salt and black pepper to taste

Skin the chicken (chopping off the knuckles and wing tips can make this easier) and remove any visible fat.

Place the bird in a large piece of aluminium foil in a roasting tin, ensuring the wings and legs are tucked in. Arrange the lemon slices over the breast and legs, tucking some into the wings.

Brush the chicken with the lemon juice and sprinkle the parsley, thyme and zest over the chicken and wrap tightly in the foil. Cook in a preheated oven at 190°C, 375°F, or Gas Mark 5 for approximately $1\frac{1}{2}$ hours.

Remove the chicken from the oven, drain off and reserve any juices. Re-cover and return to the oven for a further $\frac{1}{2}$ hour.

Remove any fat from the reserved juices. Add enough water to the juices to make up to approximately 8 fl oz (200 ml) and mix with cornflour. Season to taste. Bring to the boil to thicken, stirring continuously.

Slice the chicken and arrange on a serving dish. Pour the herby lemon sauce over.

Serve with Dry-roast Potatoes (page 175) and Savoury Carrots (page 175).

The lemon sauce adds a really fresh flavour to the chicken and cooking enclosed in foil keeps all the juices in.

Chicken Korma

(Serves 4)

$1\frac{1}{2}$ lb (600 g) chicken breast
1 medium onion, peeled and sliced
1 x $1\frac{1}{2}$ oz (32 g) sachet Schwartz World Cuisine
Mix for Chicken Korma
13 fl oz (325 ml) semi-skimmed or skimmed milk (in
addition to allowance)

Cut the chicken into cubes and dry-fry together with the onion in a non-stick frying pan. Add the contents of the chicken korma sachet and cook for 1 minute, stirring continuously. Stir in the milk and bring to the boil. Simmer gently uncovered for 20–25 minutes or until the chicken is tender, stirring occasionally.

Alternatively place the cubed chicken and sliced onion in a microwave dish. Cover and cook on *high* for 6 minutes, stirring once. Blend the contents of the chicken korma sachet in 8 fl oz (200 ml) of the milk. Pour over the chicken, cover and cook on *high* for 6 minutes or until the chicken is tender.

Serve with boiled brown rice (2 oz/50 g [dry weight] per person).

Chicken Madras

(Serves 4)

1 medium onion, peeled and chopped
1 clove garlic, peeled and crushed
1 lb (400 g) chicken or 4 chicken breasts, skinned, boned and chopped
1 tsp each of cumin, coriander, turmeric, garam masala and madras curry powder
$^1/_2$ tsp chilli (or more if you prefer hotter dishes)
salt and black pepper to taste
1 x 8 oz (200 g) can chopped tomatoes
1 carrot, trimmed, scraped and cut into thin sticks
4 oz (100 g) mushrooms, sliced
2 oz (50 g) frozen peas
1 level tbsp cornflour
1 tbsp mango chutney
1 carton low-fat natural yogurt

Dry-fry the onion and garlic in a non-stick frying pan. Cook gently for 10 minutes. Add the chicken, spices and seasoning and fry until the spices are soaked in. Cook for a further 2 minutes and add the tomatoes. Cover and cook for 30 minutes, stirring occasionally.

Add the carrot, mushrooms and peas and simmer for a further 20 minutes.

Mix the cornflour with water and stir into the ingredients in the pan. Add the mango chutney. Bring back to the boil then remove from heat, and stir in the yogurt.

Garnish with finely chopped onions, tomatoes and cucumber, and serve immediately with boiled rice (2 oz/50 g [dry weight] per person).

Chicken and Mushroom Bake

(Serves 2)

3 medium-sized potatoes
6 oz (150 g) cooked chicken, diced
1 clove garlic, thinly sliced
1 oz (25 g) frozen peas
2 spring onions, finely chopped
black pepper to taste
3 oz (75 g) mushrooms, sliced
1 packet Batchelors Slim a Soup
(Chicken and Sweetcorn or Chicken and Mushroom)

Scrub the potatoes and boil with the skins on until cooked.

Meanwhile, place the chicken in the bottom of a casserole dish. Add the garlic, frozen peas and spring onions to the chicken. Season with black pepper. Lay the mushrooms over the top of the chicken.

Make up the Slim a Soup a little thicker than normal in a cup, removing any croûtons. Reserve a quarter of the soup mix and pour the remainder into the casserole.

Drain and slice the potatoes and lay them on top of the casserole mixture. Spoon the remaining soup over the sliced potatoes.

Bake uncovered in a preheated oven at 190°C, 375°F, or Gas Mark 5 for 15 minutes. Serve with unlimited vegetables.

Chicken Paprika

(Serves 4)

1 lb (400 g) boneless chicken
$^1/_2$ oz (12.5 g) plain flour
1 tbsp paprika
1 onion, peeled and sliced
1 small green pepper, deseeded and sliced
1 clove garlic, peeled and crushed
$^1/_2$ pint/10 fl oz (250 ml) semi-skimmed or skimmed milk (in addition to allowance)
1 tbsp tomato purée
salt and black pepper to taste
4 oz (100 g) mushrooms, sliced
2 oz (50 g) frozen peas
2 oz (50 g) sweetcorn, canned or frozen
low-fat natural yogurt and paprika to garnish

Cut the chicken into $^3/_4$ inch (2 cm) pieces.

Mix the flour and paprika together and use to coat the chicken pieces.

Place the chicken in a large saucepan and add the onion, green pepper and garlic. Mix well. Stir in the milk and tomato purée. Bring to the boil. Season with salt and pepper. Add the mushrooms. Cover and simmer for 35 minutes, stirring occasionally. Add the peas and sweetcorn to the chicken and cook for a further 10 minutes. Remove from the heat. Top with a swirl of yogurt and sprinkle with paprika.

Serve on a bed of boiled brown rice. Allow 2 oz/50 g (dry weight) per person.

Chicken Provençale with Peppers and Onions

(Serves 4)

16 oz (400 g) chicken breast, boned and skinned
1 medium onion, peeled and chopped
1 x 14$^1/_2$ oz (360 g) jar Uncle Ben's Sauce Provençale with Peppers and Onions

Chop the chicken and dry-fry with the onion in a non-stick frying pan. When almost cooked, add the provençale sauce and cook for a further 5 minutes.

Serve with boiled brown rice (2 oz/50 g [dry weight] per person).

Chicken Risotto

(Serves 2)

4 oz (100 g) [dry weight] long-grain brown rice
1 small onion, peeled and chopped
1 stick celery, chopped
1 x 8 oz (200 g) can chopped tomatoes in herbs
1 chicken stock cube dissolved in $^3/_4$ pint (375 ml)
boiling water
1 tsp dried mixed herbs
1 x 8 oz (200 g) cooked chicken
or turkey fillets, cut into strips
4 oz (100 g) mushrooms, chopped
1 red pepper, deseeded and chopped
1 oz (25 g) frozen peas

Place the rice, onion, celery, tomatoes, chicken stock and herbs in a large frying pan and simmer, with the lid on, for 20–25 minutes.

Add the chicken or turkey, mushrooms, pepper and peas and simmer gently for a further 15 minutes, stirring occasionally. Add a little extra water if needed. All the water should be absorbed and the rice soft when cooked.

Serve with additional green vegetables.

Chilli Chicken

(Serves 2)

1 medium onion, peeled and finely chopped
2 cloves garlic, peeled and crushed
2 fresh green chillies, crushed or finely chopped
(including seeds)
8 oz (200 g) chicken breast, all skin removed
1 x 8 oz (200 g) can chopped tomatoes
1 tbsp tomato purée
good squeeze lemon or lime juice
1 tsp dried oregano
salt to taste
sugar to taste
2 tbsp low-fat fromage frais

Dry-fry the onion, garlic and chillies until softened. Add 1 tablespoon of water if the mixture begins to stick. Add the chicken and continue stirring for 4–5 minutes.

Stir in the tomatoes, tomato purée, lemon or lime juice and oregano. Bring to the boil, reduce the heat, then simmer for 20 minutes. Add the salt and sugar to taste.

Remove from the heat and stir in the fromage frais. Serve immediately with boiled brown rice (2 oz/50 g [dry weight] per person) and unlimited green salad.

Chinese Chicken with Pineapple

(Serves 4)

$1^1/_2$ lb (600 g) chicken breast, skinned
1 medium onion, peeled and chopped
1 x 18 oz (450 g) jar Del Monte Quality Chinese
with Pineapple Sauce

Chop the chicken into bite size pieces and dry-fry with the onion in a non-stick frying pan. When almost cooked, add the sauce and cook for a further 5 minutes.

Serve with boiled brown rice (2 oz/50 g [dry weight] per person).

Coq au Vin

(Serves 4)

4 x 6 oz (150 g) chicken breasts, boned and skinned
2 medium onions, peeled and sliced
4 oz (100 g) mushrooms, sliced
1 x 2 oz (50 g) sachet Colman's Coq au Vin
Casserole Mix

Place the chicken breasts, onions and mushrooms into an ovenproof dish. Mix the contents of the casserole mix sachet with $^3/_4$ pint/15 fl oz (475 ml) water and stir into the dish. Cover and cook in a preheated oven at 180°C, 350°F, or Gas Mark 4 for about $1^1/_2$ hours or until the chicken is tender.

Serve with unlimited potatoes and vegetables.

Spiced Turkey

(Serves 4)

1 large onion, peeled and sliced
2 cloves garlic, peeled and crushed
1 tbsp curry powder, or to taste
12 oz (300 g) potatoes
12 oz (300 g) cooked turkey
1 pint/20 fl oz (500 ml) semi-skimmed or skimmed
milk (in addition to allowance)
1 tbsp tomato purée
8 oz (200 g) cabbage, shredded

Dry-fry the onion and garlic in a non-stick frying pan for 5 minutes. Stir in the curry powder and cook for 2 minutes on a gentle heat. Cut the potatoes into $^1/_2$ inch (1 cm) cubes (do not peel). Add the potatoes, turkey, milk and tomato purée to the onion mixture. Bring to the boil, cover and simmer for 15 minutes or until the potatoes are cooked.

Add the shredded cabbage to the pan. Cook for 5 minutes, uncovered.

Stir-fry Chicken in Black Bean Sauce

(Serves 4)

16 oz (400 g) chicken breast, skinned
1 medium onion, peeled and chopped
1 x $14^1/_2$ oz (360 g) jar Uncle Ben's Black Bean with
Crispy Vegetables Stir-fry Sauce

Chop the chicken into bite-size pieces and dry-fry together with the onion in a non-stick frying pan. When almost cooked, add the sauce and cook for a further 5 minutes.

Serve with boiled brown rice (2 oz/50 g [dry weight] per person).

Tandoori Chicken Thatch

(Serves 4)

1 lb (400 g) potatoes, peeled
1 tbsp tandoori paste
1 tbsp low-fat natural yogurt
4 x 5 oz (125 g) chicken breasts, skinned
1 egg, beaten
1 tsp mixed herbs

Place the potatoes in a saucepan with enough cold water to cover, and par-boil for 8 minutes. Drain and leave to go cold.

Mix the tandoori paste and yogurt together. Flatten the chicken breasts gently with a rolling pin. Spread the tandoori mixture in a thin layer on the inner side of each and leave to marinate for half an hour.

Scrape off any excess marinade from the chicken, roll up, secure with cocktail sticks and place on a lightly greased baking sheet.

Coarsely grate the potatoes and mix with enough egg to moisten. Stir in the herbs and mould the potatoes around the chicken breasts.

Bake in a preheated oven at 200°C, 400°F, or Gas Mark 6 for 40–45 minutes until the potato is golden and the chicken is tender.

Serve with Ratatouille (page 175).

Tarragon Chicken
(Serves 4)

4 skinless chicken fillets
1 medium onion, peeled and chopped
12 button mushrooms, halved
1 chicken stock cube dissolved in
$^1/_4$ pint/5 fl oz (125 ml) boiling water
3 tsp tarragon
salt and black pepper to taste
1 tbsp cornflour
2 tbsp low-fat natural yogurt
50 g (2 oz) seedless green grapes, halved

Place the chicken, onion, mushrooms, stock, tarragon and seasoning into a shallow covered casserole dish and cook in a preheated oven at 180°C, 350°F, or Gas Mark 4 for approximately 1 hour, ensuring the chicken is cooked thoroughly.

Blend the cornflour with a little water and stir into the casserole mixture. Return to the oven for 5 minutes to thicken.

Mix in the yogurt and grapes and serve immediately.

Serve with potatoes and unlimited green vegetables.

Tarragon Chicken Salad
(Serves 4)

12 oz (300 g) cooked chicken,
cut into bite-sized pieces
1 bunch spring onions, chopped
8 oz (200 g) black grapes, halved, with pips removed
10 oz (250 g) low-fat fromage frais or natural yogurt
1 tbsp fresh or 1 tsp dried tarragon
salt and black pepper to taste
lemon juice
watercress to garnish

Place the chicken, spring onions and grapes in a large bowl. Mix the fromage frais or yogurt with the tarragon. Season with salt, lots of black pepper and lemon juice to taste. Pour the dressing over the chicken and vegetables and mix well.

To serve, arrange the watercress around the edge of the dish and pile the chicken mixture in the centre.

Spicy Sweet and Sour Chicken or Pork with Crispy Vegetables
(Serves 2)

12 oz (300 g) chicken breast or pork
1 medium onion, peeled and chopped
1 x 14$^1/_2$ oz (360 g) jar Uncle Ben's Extra Spicy Stir-fry Sweet and Sour Sauce with Crispy Vegetables

Chop the chicken or pork and dry-fry with the onion in a non-stick frying pan. When almost cooked, add the sweet and sour sauce and cook for a further 5 minutes.

Serve with boiled brown rice (2 oz/50 g [dry weight] per person).

Sweet and Sour Chicken or Prawns with Crispy Vegetables
(Serves 4)

16 oz (400 g) chicken breast, chopped,
or 8 oz (200 g) cooked prawns
1 medium onion, peeled and chopped
1 x 14$^1/_2$ oz (360 g) jar Uncle Ben's Sweet and Sour Stir-fry Sauce with Crispy Vegetables

If using chicken, dry-fry the chicken with the onion in a non-stick frying pan. When almost cooked, add the sweet and sour sauce and cook for a further 5 minutes. If using prawns, dry-fry the onion, then add the prawns and the sweet and sour sauce and cook for a further 5 minutes.

Serve with boiled brown rice (2 oz/50 g [dry weight] per person).

Sweet and Sour Pork
(Serves 4)

12 oz (300 g) lean pork fillet, thinly sliced into strips
1 small onion, peeled and finely chopped
1 carrot, trimmed, scraped and sliced into julienne strips
$^1/_2$ green pepper, deseeded and finely chopped
$^1/_2$ red pepper, deseeded and finely chopped
8 oz (200 g) bean sprouts, washed and drained
4 oz (100 g) mushrooms, sliced or chopped
small can pineapple chunks in natural juice
2 tbsp malt vinegar
2 tbsp tomato purée
pinch salt
1 tsp honey
1 tbsp soy sauce

Dry-stir-fry pork fillet in a wok or large saucepan for 5 minutes. Add the vegetables in the order listed in the ingredients, cooking each for 30 seconds before adding the next.

Drain the pineapple, reserving the juice, and stir into the pork mixture. Mix the pineapple juice with the vinegar, tomato purée, salt, honey and soy sauce and add to the pork mixture, continuing to stir for a few more minutes until pork is well cooked.

Serve on a bed of plain boiled rice. Allow 2 oz/50 g (dry weight) per person.

Pork Casserole

(Serves 4)

16 oz (400 g) pork, cut into cubes
2 medium onions, peeled and sliced
2 large carrots, trimmed, scraped and sliced
4 oz (100 g) frozen green beans
1 x 1¹/₂ oz (40 g) sachet Colman's Traditional Pork
Casserole Mix

Place the pork into an ovenproof dish. Add the onions, carrots and green beans.

Mix the contents of the casserole mix sachet with ³/₄ pint/15 fl oz (375 ml) water and stir into the dish. Cover and cook in a preheated oven at 180°C, 350°F, or Gas Mark 4 for about 1¹/₂ hours or until the pork is tender.

Serve with unlimited vegetables and potatoes.

Tasty Pork with Pasta

(Serves 4)

12 oz (300 g) pork, sliced into thin strips
1 small onion, peeled and sliced
4 oz (100 g) mushrooms, sliced
1 stick celery, sliced
1 small green pepper, deseeded and cut into strips
1 small red pepper, deseeded and cut into strips
1 small can pineapple cubes in natural juice
¹/₄ pint/5 fl oz (125 ml) tomato juice
1 tbsp white wine vinegar
salt and black pepper to taste
1 oz (25 g) cornflour

Dry-fry the pork and onion in a large non-stick frying pan until the pork is sealed and the onion soft. Add the mushrooms, celery, peppers and pineapple (including the juice), tomato juice and wine vinegar. Season to taste. Bring to the boil and simmer gently for 30 minutes.

Mix the cornflour with a little water and add to the pan, stirring until sauce is thickened.

Serve with cooked pasta (2 oz/50 g [dry weight] per person).

Soufflé Potato and Ham Bake

(Serves 4)

8 oz (200 g) broccoli, cut into spears and blanched
1¹/₄ lb (500 g) potatoes, peeled and cooked
2 tbsp semi-skimmed or skimmed milk (in addition
to allowance)
1 tbsp low-fat natural yogurt
1 oz (25 g) plain flour
salt and black pepper to taste
3 eggs, separated
6 spring onions, chopped
6 oz (150 g) smoked ham, chopped
1 tbsp fresh chives, chopped
¹/₂ tsp paprika

Place the broccoli in the base of a lightly greased 7 inch (18 cm) soufflé dish.

Mash the potatoes with the milk and yogurt. Work in the flour and season well. Stir in the egg yolks, spring onions, ham and chives.

Whisk the egg whites until they form soft peaks, then gently but thoroughly fold into the potato mixture.

Spread the mixture on top of the broccoli and sprinkle with paprika. Bake in a preheated oven at 200°C, 400°F, or Gas Mark 6 for 25 minutes or until well risen and golden brown.

Serve immediately with fresh vegetables.

FISH

Baked Haddock

(Serves 4)

4 x 6 oz (150 g) haddock fillets, boned and skinned
8 spring onions, chopped
4 oz (100 g) button mushrooms, sliced
1 tbsp cornflour
¹/₂ pint/10 fl oz (250 ml) semi-skimmed
or skimmed milk (in addition to allowance)
1 clove garlic, crushed
2 tsp chopped fresh mint
(use dried if fresh not available)
1 tbsp lemon juice
salt and black pepper to taste

Place the haddock fillets in a shallow ovenproof dish. Sprinkle the spring onions and mushrooms over the fish.

Blend the cornflour with 2 tablespoons of the milk in a saucepan, then add the remaining milk, garlic, mint and lemon juice. Mix well and season with salt and pepper. Bring to the boil, stirring continuously. Pour the sauce over the fish.

Cover with foil, and bake in a preheated oven at 180°C, 350°F, or Gas Mark 4 for about 20 minutes.

Serve with unlimited vegetables and potatoes.

Cod, Bacon, Cheese and Onion Bake

(Serves 1)

6 oz (150 g) cod fillet, washed and dried
salt and black pepper to taste
2 tsp lemon or lime juice
1 rasher lean bacon, trimmed and cut into strips
¹/₂ small onion, peeled and finely chopped
1 tbsp low-fat natural yogurt
¹/₂ oz (12.5 g) low-fat Cheddar cheese, grated
chopped fresh parsley to garnish

Sprinkle the fish with salt, pepper and a little lemon or lime juice.

Line a grill pan with aluminium foil and place under a hot grill until the foil is hot.

Place the fish on the hot foil, and grill on *high* for 1–2 minutes. Reduce the heat and continue to cook for a further 2–3 minutes until the fish is just cooked.

Meanwhile dry-fry the bacon and onion in a non-stick pan until the bacon is crisp and the onion soft. Drain on kitchen paper to remove any traces of fat. Mix with the yogurt.

Place the fish on a heatproof, preheated dish. Cover with the yogurt mixture and top with the grated cheese. Place under the grill for a further 2 minutes until the cheese has melted.

Garnish with parsley and serve with a jacket potato and unlimited vegetables.

Note: For the purposes of the flavour a small amount of low-fat Cheddar cheese is permitted in this recipe.

Cod in Parsley Sauce

(Serves 1)

4 oz (100 g) cod
2 tsp cornflour
$1/4$ pint/5 fl oz (125 ml) semi-skimmed
or skimmed milk (in addition to allowance)
chopped fresh parsley to taste

Place the cod in a little of the milk in a covered saucepan and simmer gently for 10–15 minutes. Drain.

In a saucepan blend the cornflour with a little of the remaining milk to form a smooth paste. Heat gently, adding the rest of the milk and stirring continuously. Add the parsley just before serving.

Serve the fish, topped with the sauce, with unlimited vegetables and potatoes.

Cullercoats Pie

(Serves 4)

$1^1/2$ lb (600 g) potatoes, peeled and chopped
2 tbsp virtually fat-free fromage frais
1 lb (400 g) fish fillets, any combination of haddock,
cod, coley, etc.
1 tsp lemon juice
1 bay leaf
black pepper to taste
1 large leek, sliced
1 clove garlic, peeled and crushed
1 tsp dried oregano
pinch chilli powder
4 oz (100 g) mushrooms, sliced
1 x 8 oz (200 g) can chopped tomatoes
4 oz (100 g) peeled prawns
salt to taste

Cook the potatoes in boiling, salted water, for 15–20 minutes until just soft. Drain and mash with the fromage frais.

Place the fish in a saucepan with the lemon juice, bay leaf, pepper and approximately 6 fl oz (150 ml) water. Cover and poach for about 10 minutes until the fish is just flaking.

Remove the fish from the pan, drain and flake, removing the skin and bones. Strain the fish stock, return it to the pan and boil gently to reduce to about $1/4$ pint/5 fl oz (125 ml).

Add the leek, garlic, herbs and chilli to the fish stock and boil, covered, for 5 minutes. Remove the lid, stir in the mushrooms and continue to cook until the liquid is almost gone.

Add the chopped tomatoes and heat through.

Remove from heat, stir in the flaked fish and prawns, and season to taste. Place in a pie dish and pipe the mashed potato mixture around the edge.

Bake in a preheated oven at 220°C, 425°F, or Gas Mark 7 for 30 minutes or until the potato is browned.

Serve with unlimited green vegetables.

Mediterranean Tuna Lasagne

(Serves 4)

1 aubergine
1 x 16 oz (400 g) can chopped tomatoes
(preferably with added herbs or garlic)
3 courgettes or 1 small marrow, wiped and sliced
2 large onions, peeled and chopped
2 red peppers, deseeded and sliced
2–3 cloves garlic, peeled and crushed
2 tsp oregano
2 tsp basil
1 tsp chilli powder (a little more if you like it hot)
salt and black pepper to taste
1 x 16 oz (400 g) can tuna in brine
8 oz (200 g) lasagne verdi (no pre-cooking type)
$1/4$ pint/5 fl oz (125 ml) water

Wipe and slice the aubergine, sprinkle with salt and spread on a plate. Leave for 20 minutes. Transfer to a colander and rinse well in cold water.

Place the tomatoes in a large saucepan, bring to the boil and add the rinsed aubergine, courgettes or marrow, onions and peppers together with the garlic, herbs, chilli powder and seasoning.

Simmer for approximately 40 minutes until all vegetables are well cooked, stirring occasionally. Drain the tuna and mix with the vegetables.

Place a layer of the vegetable mixture on the base of a casserole dish, followed by a layer of lasagne (do not use too much lasagne). Continue layering, ending with a thick layer of vegetable mixture on the top. Ensure all the lasagne is covered. Finally, pour the water over to add moisture.

Cook in a preheated oven at 190°C, 375°F, or Gas Mark 5 for 45–50 minutes.

Serve with unlimited green salad.

Trout Parcels with Dill Sauce

(Serves 4)

4 sheets of greaseproof paper approximately
12 inches (30 cm) square
4 oz (100 g) carrots, trimmed, scraped and
cut into matchstick pieces
4 oz (100 g) leeks, cut into matchstick pieces
4 cloves garlic, peeled and crushed
4 sprigs fresh rosemary
4 small sprigs fresh dill
4 x 8 oz (200 g) trout, heads removed
4 tbsp lemon juice

Sauce
$1/2$ pint/10 fl oz (250 ml) semi-skimmed
or skimmed milk (in addition to allowance)
1 tbsp cornflour
1 clove garlic, crushed (optional)
2 tsp dill and rosemary

Lay the sheets of greaseproof paper on a large baking sheet. Place a quarter of the carrots and leeks in the centre of each.

Place a clove of garlic, a sprig of rosemary and one of dill into each trout. Lay the trout on the carrots and leeks. Spoon 1 tablespoon of lemon juice over each. Fold over the edges of each paper to enclose the trout and make neat parcels. Bake in a preheated oven at 180°C, 350°F, or Gas Mark 4 for 20 minutes.

Meanwhile, make the sauce. Blend the milk, cornflour, garlic and herbs together. Bring to the boil, stirring continuously. Serve the sauce with the fish.

Serve with potatoes and additional vegetables.

Trout and Spinach Salad

(Serves 4)

10 oz (250 g) trout, cooked and roughly flaked
4 oz (100 g) small green beans, topped, tailed,
blanched and halved
6 oz (150 g) spinach leaves, stalked and shredded
1 medium ruby grapefruit, segmented, juice reserved
10 oz (250 g) new potatoes, well scrubbed,
cooked and halved
salt and black pepper to taste
4 tbsp low-fat fromage frais
watercress sprigs to garnish

Place the flaked trout, green beans, spinach, grapefruit segments and new potatoes in a bowl. Season and mix together.

Beat together the fromage frais and 3 tablespoons of reserved grapefruit juice. Pour over the salad. Toss gently to coat all the ingredients.

Garnish with watercress and serve on a mixed green salad with 1 slice (1 oz/25 g) wholemeal or granary bread per person.

Tuna, Mushroom and Pasta Serenade

(Serves 4–6)

4 oz (100 g) mushrooms, sliced
$3/4$ pint/15 fl oz (375 ml) semi-skimmed or skimmed
milk (in addition to allowance)
salt and black pepper to taste
pinch mixed herbs
1 bay leaf
$1/2$ chicken stock cube
pinch dried parsley (or chopped fresh)
8 oz (200 g) tricolour pasta
2 oz (50 g) sweetcorn, canned or frozen
2 oz (50 g) peas, canned or frozen
1 x 8 oz (200 g) can tuna in brine, drained
2 rounded tsp cornflour

Place the mushrooms, milk (reserving just a little for thickening), seasoning, herbs, bay leaf, stock cube and

parsley into a saucepan. Bring to the boil, simmer for 5 minutes, then leave to infuse for 30 minutes with the lid on.

Cook the pasta in salted water, adding the sweetcorn and peas 5 minutes before the end of cooking time. Drain well. Break up the tuna and add to the pasta.

Mix the cornflour in cold milk and blend into the mushroom sauce mix. Remove the bay leaf. Bring to the boil to thicken, then combine with the pasta and tuna.

Serve with green vegetables or salad.

Tuna and Sweetcorn Cakes

(Serves 4)

$1^1/2$ lb (600 g) potatoes, peeled and cooked
1 tbsp low-fat fromage frais
salt and black pepper to taste
1 x 8 oz (200 g) can tuna in brine, drained
1 x 8 oz (200 g) can sweetcorn, drained
1 small onion, peeled and finely chopped
2 tbsp reduced-oil salad dressing
$1/2$ tsp mixed herbs
1 tbsp fresh parsley, chopped
1 egg, beaten
4 oz (100 g) fresh granary breadcrumbs

Mash the potatoes well with the low-fat fromage frais, and season.

Place the tuna, sweetcorn and onion in a bowl and stir in the reduced-oil salad dressing, mixed herbs and parsley. Season well.

On a floured board take a quarter of the potato mixture, flatten, and place a large tablespoon of the fish mixture in the centre. Mould the potato mixture around the fish until the fish is completely covered and sealed. Flatten, brush well with the beaten egg, and coat with the breadcrumbs. Repeat with the remaining mixture to make a further 3 cakes.

Grill for 20 minutes turning frequently until crisp and golden brown.

Serve with a green salad.

Tuna Pasta with Tomatoes

(Serves 4)

1 medium onion, peeled and chopped
2 cloves garlic, peeled and crushed
1 x 14 oz (350 g) can chopped tomatoes
1 tbsp tomato purée
$1/4$ pint/5 fl oz (125 ml) white wine
(use from daily allowance)
8 oz (200 g) [dry weight] wholewheat pasta shapes
1 x 8 oz (200 g) can tuna chunks in brine, drained
2 tsp dried basil or few sprigs fresh basil
salt and black pepper to taste

Dry-fry the onions and garlic in a large non-stick frying pan, being careful not to let them burn. Add the tomatoes, purée and wine, and stir well. Bring to the boil, reduce the heat and simmer for 10–15 minutes.

Boil the pasta according to the instructions on the packet (8–10 minutes).

Add the drained tuna, basil and seasoning to the sauce and stir in well until the tuna is warmed through.

Drain the pasta and return to the pan. Add the tuna mixture and gently mix together.

Serve immediately with a green salad.

VEGETARIAN

Blackeye Bean Casserole

(Serves 2)

2 oz (50 g) blackeye beans
2 oz (50 g) onion, peeled and diced
6 oz (150 g) mushrooms, sliced
4 oz (100 g) celery, cut into thin strips
3 oz (75 g) carrots, trimmed, scraped and cut into
thin strips
2 oz (50 g) water chestnuts, thinly sliced
$1/2$ tsp chilli powder
$1/2$ tsp grated fresh ginger or $1/2$ tsp ground ginger
1 clove garlic, peeled and crushed
$1/2$ oz (12.5 g) cornflour
1 tbsp soy sauce
$1/4$ pint/5 fl oz (125 ml) vegetable stock
black pepper to taste

Cook the blackeye beans in plenty of water for 30–35 minutes, by bringing to the boil and then simmering in a covered saucepan.

Gently heat the vegetables, chilli, ginger and garlic in a little stock for 10 minutes. Mix the cornflour and soy sauce in a separate pan with a little of the remaining stock and then stir in the rest of the stock. Add this mixture to the vegetables and then add the drained blackeye beans. Simmer for 8–10 minutes and season to taste.

Serve on a bed of boiled brown rice (2 oz/50 g [dry weight] per person).

Broccoli Delight

(Serves 4)

1 lb (400 g) frozen broccoli florets

Flan case
2 oz (50 g) oats
2 oz (50 g) wholewheat flour
1 tsp baking powder
1 tsp dried oregano
1 clove garlic, peeled and crushed
salt and black pepper to taste
2 egg whites
3 fl oz (75 ml) semi-skimmed or skimmed milk
(in addition to allowance)

Topping
3 oz (75 g) low-fat Cheddar cheese, grated
3 fl oz (75 ml) semi-skimmed or skimmed milk (in addition to allowance)
2 egg whites
1 small onion, peeled and finely chopped
1 clove garlic, peeled and crushed
salt and pepper to taste

Very lightly grease or spray with non-stick cooking spray an 8 in (20 cm) baking tin.

Cook the broccoli in boiling salted water until just soft. Drain well.

To prepare the flan case
In a large bowl combine all the dry crust ingredients and spices. Mix well. In a separate small bowl, mix the egg whites and milk together and beat until well blended. Add this to the dry mixture, stirring until all the ingredients are moistened. Spread this mixture evenly in the prepared baking tin.

Place the drained broccoli on top of the crust and press down firmly with the back of a spoon so that it fits well into the flan case.

To prepare the topping
Sprinkle the grated cheese over the broccoli.

Combine all the remaining ingredients (milk, egg whites, onion, garlic, salt and pepper) in a blender or food processor and blend until smooth. Pour over the broccoli and cheese.

Bake uncovered in a preheated oven at 180°C, 350°F, or Gas Mark 4 for 30 minutes. Cut into squares and serve hot with additional vegetables or salad.

Cabbage and Leek Bake

(Serves 2)

1 medium white cabbage, thinly sliced
2 large leeks, thinly sliced
salt and black pepper to taste
8 oz (200 g) low-fat fromage frais
3 medium tomatoes, sliced
6 oz (150 g) fresh breadcrumbs

Arrange the sliced cabbage and leeks in the base of a microwave dish. Cover with cling film and cook in a microwave on *full* power for 5 minutes until just cooked. Remove cling film and season well. Alternatively, place the cabbage and leeks in a saucepan with a little water. Cover with a lid and boil for 5 minutes. Drain, and place in an ovenproof dish. Season well.

Cover with the fromage frais, sliced tomatoes and breadcrumbs.

Bake in a preheated oven at 190°C, 375°F, or Gas Mark 5 for approximately 30 minutes until breadcrumbs are nicely browned.

Serve with additional vegetables if desired.

Note: This is rather like a vegetable crumble – the fromage frais gives it a rich texture.

Chickpea and Fennel Casserole

(Serves 2)

3 oz (75 g) cooked chickpeas
1 oz (25 g) bulgar wheat
6 oz (150 g) celery, diced
2 tsp crushed fennel seeds
1 clove garlic, peeled and crushed
$^1/_2$ pint/10 fl oz (250 ml) vegetable stock
6 oz (150 g) whole green beans, chopped
2 tbsp soy sauce
salt and black pepper to taste
2 tbsp chopped fresh mint, to garnish

Cook the chickpeas, bulgar wheat, celery, fennel and garlic gently in a little stock for about 5 minutes. Add the remaining ingredients, excluding the mint, and simmer for 20 minutes.

Garnish with fresh mint and serve with boiled brown rice (2 oz/50 g [dry weight] per person) and unlimited vegetables.

Curried Chickpeas

(Serves 4)

2 tsp pure sunflower oil
1 onion, peeled and sliced
1 tbsp mild curry powder
1 tbsp wholemeal flour
1 x 14 oz (350 g) can chickpeas, drained
1 x 8 oz (200 g) can pineapple pieces, in natural juice, drained
3 oz (75 g) raisins
2 oz (50 g) ground almonds (optional)
$^1/_2$ pint/10 fl oz (250 ml) semi-skimmed or skimmed milk (in addition to allowance)
salt to taste
1 eating apple
1 tbsp lemon juice

Heat the oil in a saucepan and fry the onion until softened.

Stir in the curry powder and flour and cook on a gentle heat for 2 minutes.

Add the chickpeas and mix to coat with curry mixture. Stir in the pineapple, raisins, ground almonds (if desired) and milk. Season, and bring to the boil. Cover and simmer for 20 minutes.

Core the apple and chop into $^1/_2$ inch (1 cm) pieces. Add to the curry mixture, then add the lemon juice and cook for 5 minutes.

Serve with boiled brown rice. Allow 2 oz/50 g (dry weight) per person.

Mixed Bean Hotpot
(Serves 4)

1 lb (400 g) canned beans, drained
and rinsed (see below)
4 oz (100 g) green beans
1 x 16 oz (400 g) can tomatoes
1 tbsp tomato purée
1 clove garlic, peeled and crushed
1 tsp mixed herbs
salt and black pepper to taste
1 lb (400 g) potatoes, par-boiled
4 oz (100 g) half-fat Cheddar type cheese, grated

Place the beans in an ovenproof casserole dish. Mix together the remaining ingredients except the potatoes and cheese. Pour over the beans and mix well.

Thinly slice the par-boiled potatoes and lay the sliced potatoes on top of the bean mixture. Sprinkle with the grated cheese. Cook in a preheated oven at 160°C, 325°F, or Gas Mark 3 for 1 hour until the potatoes are cooked.

Serve with additional vegetables or salad.

Note: Use a selection of beans such as red or white kidney beans, borlotti beans, butter beans, pinto beans, blackeye beans, flageolet beans.

Quorn Bolognese
(Serves 1)

1 small onion, peeled and chopped
7 oz (175 g) mixed Quorn
1 clove garlic, peeled and crushed
$^1/_2$ tsp dried mixed herbs
3 fl oz (75 ml) red wine
1 tsp red pesto
1 tbsp tomato purée
1 x 7 oz (175 g) can chopped tomatoes
1 tsp sugar
salt and black pepper to taste

Dry-fry the onion in a non-stick frying pan until soft. Add the Quorn, crushed garlic, dried herbs plus 1 tablespoon of the red wine, and continue to fry for 3 minutes. Add the red pesto, tomato purée and chopped tomatoes, and stir well. Add the remaining red wine and sugar, bring to the boil and simmer for 20 minutes.

Season to taste, and serve with spaghetti (allow 2 oz/50 g [dry weight] per person).

Spiced Bean Casserole
(Serves 2)

2 oz (50 g) onion, chopped
1 x 8 oz (200 g) can tomatoes
$^3/_4$ tsp mild chilli powder
$^1/_2$ tsp tomato purée
1 oz (25 g) wholemeal flour
$^1/_4$ pint/5 fl oz (125 ml) vegetable stock
$^1/_2$ tsp garlic granules
pinch salt
4 oz (100 g) courgettes, sliced
6 oz (150 g) red and green peppers,
deseeded and sliced
1 x 8 oz (200 g) can red kidney beans,
washed and drained
1 x 8 oz (200 g) can haricot beans,
washed and drained
4 oz (100 g) sweetcorn

Dry-fry the onion in a non-stick frying pan until soft. Add the tomatoes, mild chilli powder, tomato purée and wholemeal flour and mix well.

Gradually add the vegetable stock together with the garlic granules, salt, sliced courgettes and peppers. Add the drained beans and sweetcorn and bring to the boil. Cover and simmer for 10–12 minutes or until vegetables are tender.

Serve with mashed potatoes or boiled brown rice. Allow 2 oz/50 g (dry weight) rice per person.

Spicy Chickpea Casserole
(Serves 4)

8 oz (200 g) [dry weight] chickpeas
(soaked overnight)
1 medium–large onion, peeled and chopped
1 medium-sized can tomatoes
$^1/_2$ tsp coriander
2 heaped tsp cumin seeds (or 1 tsp ground cumin)
$^1/_2$–1 tsp chilli powder
salt and black pepper to taste
8 oz (200 g) mushrooms, sliced

Fast-boil the chickpeas for 10 minutes and then simmer for a further 20–25 minutes until fairly soft.

Meanwhile, place the onion and tomatoes into a medium saucepan, and mix in the coriander, cumin, chilli and seasoning. Bring to the boil and simmer gently for 10 minutes.

When the chickpeas are almost cooked, drain, rinse with boiling water and stir into the tomato mixture. Add the mushrooms and simmer for a further 5 minutes.

Serve with boiled brown rice (2 oz/50 g [dry weight] per person) and unlimited vegetables.

Stuffed Marrow
(Serves 4)

$1^1/_2$ lb (600 g) assorted vegetables, chopped
1 oz (25 g) onion, peeled and chopped
2 cloves garlic, peeled and crushed
2 tbsp tomato purée
2 tsp chopped fresh rosemary or 1 tsp dried rosemary
salt and black pepper to taste
4 oz (100 g) [dry weight] long-grain brown rice
1 medium-sized marrow, skinned,
cut lengthways and deseeded

In a saucepan cook the vegetables, onion, garlic, tomato purée and rosemary in a little water seasoned with salt and pepper. Simmer until tender. Remove from the heat, place in a container and, if possible, leave overnight.

Cook the rice in a saucepan of boiling salted water until tender. Drain, and mix the rice with the vegetable mixture. Spoon into the marrow halves.

Wrap the stuffed marrow in aluminium foil and bake in a preheated oven at 200°C, 400°F, or Gas Mark 6 for 1 hour.

Stuffed Pitta Bread with Yogurt Salad

(Serves 2)

1 medium potato
1 carrot
1 small onion
$^1/_2$ tbsp sunflower oil
$^1/_2$ tsp sesame seeds
1 tsp lemon juice
$^1/_2$ cup frozen peas
$^1/_2$ cup sweetcorn
pinch haldi (turmeric powder)
$^1/_2$ tsp salt
1 green chilli, finely grated
small piece ginger, finely grated
2 small wholemeal pitta breads

Peel and chop the potato, carrot and onion into small cubes and rinse with water.

Heat the sunflower oil in a pan and add the sesame seeds. Wait until the sesame seeds have popped and then add the chopped vegetables and lemon juice. Simmer for 6–8 minutes.

Add the peas and sweetcorn. Simmer for 4–5 minutes, stirring halfway.

Add the turmeric powder, salt, green chilli and ginger. Stir gently.

Warm the pitta bread by placing it in a microwave or under a grill until it puffs up. Slit the pitta bread and place the cooked vegetables inside. Serve with Yogurt Salad (see below).

Yogurt Salad

1 radish, grated
2 lettuce leaves, chopped
$^1/_2$ tomato, chopped
1 small piece green pepper, finely chopped
1 small carrot, trimmed, scraped and grated
1 small piece cucumber, finely chopped
4 tbsp low-fat natural yogurt
$^1/_2$ tsp chilli powder

Place all the salad vegetables in a bowl and add the low-fat yogurt. Stir. Add the chilli powder and stir. Serve with the Stuffed Pitta Bread.

Tofu Burgers

(Serves 2)

16 oz (400 g) medium tofu
2 oz (50 g) oats
$^1/_2$ tsp ground cumin
1 tsp chilli powder
1 clove garlic, peeled and crushed
1 onion, peeled and very finely chopped
salt and black pepper to taste

Preheat a non-stick frying pan. Place the tofu in a large bowl and mash well with a fork. Add the remaining ingredients and mix well.

Shape the mixture into 6 burgers and place into the preheated frying pan. Cook until the burgers are brown on all sides, turning them carefully.

Serve in burger buns (1 x 2 oz/50 g bun per person) with unlimited salad.

Vegetable and Fruit Curry

(Serves 4)

1 medium onion, peeled and chopped
1 large clove garlic, peeled and crushed
1–2 green chillis (according to taste), deseeded and finely chopped
1 in (2.5 cm) piece green ginger, peeled and finely chopped
$^1/_2$ pint/10 fl oz (250 ml) vegetable stock
2 tsp garam masala
1 tsp ground coriander
1 tsp ground cumin
8 oz (200 g) green beans
12 oz (300 g) cauliflower florets
1 red pepper, deseeded and finely chopped
salt to taste
2 bananas

Using a non-stick frying pan, dry-fry the chopped onion, garlic, chillis and ginger for 5 minutes on a gentle heat, covering the pan with a lid. Add a little of the vegetable stock if the pan becomes too dry.

When the onions are soft, add 2 fl oz (50 ml) of the vegetable stock and then sprinkle in the spices and cook for a further minute, stirring continuously.

Trim the beans and cut into 1 inch (2.5 cm) lengths. Break the cauliflower into small florets. Add the beans, cauliflower and pepper to the pan and cook over a moderate heat for 2–3 minutes, stirring continuously. Pour in the remaining vegetable stock and season with salt. Cover the pan and cook gently for 10 minutes.

Peel and slice the bananas and add to the pan. Cook for a further 10 minutes or until the vegetables are tender.

Serve with boiled brown rice (2 oz/50 g [dry weight] per person) and yogurt mixed with chopped cucumber and a little mint sauce.

Vegetable Casserole
(Serves 1)

selection of vegetables (approximately
1 lb/400 g in total), chopped
4 oz (100 g) lentils, presoaked
1 tsp paprika
pinch garlic granules
1/2 pint/10 fl oz (250 ml) water or vegetable stock
salt and black pepper to taste

Place the chopped vegetables and the lentils in a casserole and sprinkle with the paprika and garlic granules. Add the stock, season to taste, and cover.

Place in a preheated oven and cook at 180°C, 350°F, or Gas Mark 4 for approximately 1 hour or until the vegetables are tender.

If a main course, serve with boiled brown rice (2 oz/50 g [dry weight] per person).

Vegetable Chilli
(Serves 4)

15 oz (375 g) can tomatoes
1 bay leaf
1 eating apple, cored and chopped
2 tsp oil-free sweet pickle
1 tsp tomato purée
1 medium onion, peeled and chopped
4 oz (100 g) broad beans
4 oz (100 g) frozen peas
4 oz (100 g) carrots, trimmed, scraped and chopped
4 oz (100 g) potatoes, peeled and chopped
1 x 8 oz (200 g) can baked beans or red kidney beans
1 tsp chilli powder
3 chillis
1 tsp garlic granules
4 fl oz (100 ml) vegetable stock

Place all the ingredients in a saucepan and cover. Simmer for 1 hour, stirring occasionally. Remove the lid and continue to cook until the liquid is reduced to a thick consistency. Raise the heat if necessary.

Serve on a bed of boiled brown rice. Allow 2 oz/50 g (dry weight) per person.

Vegetable Chop Suey
(Serves 1)

1 tbsp vegetable stock
1 large carrot, trimmed, scraped and coarsely grated
3 sticks celery, finely chopped
1 large onion, peeled and finely chopped
1 green pepper, deseeded and sliced
1 x 15 oz (375 g) can bean sprouts, drained
salt and black pepper to taste
soy sauce

Pour a little stock into a non-stick frying pan or wok. Add all the vegetables, except the bean sprouts, and stir-fry, adding more stock if required. When the vegetables are hot and partly cooked, add the drained bean sprouts. Continue to cook for 5 minutes until hot.

Serve on a bed of boiled brown rice (2 oz/50 g [dry weight] per person), with soy sauce.

Vegetable Crunch
(Serves 4)

1 medium onion, peeled and roughly chopped
1 leek, sliced
1 stick celery, chopped
6 oz (150 g) mushrooms, sliced
1 lb (400 g) potatoes, peeled and cut into large pieces
6 oz (150 g) carrots, trimmed, scraped and sliced
1/2 small cauliflower, broken into small florets
parsley sprigs and tomato lily to garnish

Sauce
1/2 pint/10 fl oz (250 ml) semi-skimmed or skimmed milk (in addition to allowance)
2 tsp cornflour
salt and black pepper to taste
2 tbsp fresh parsley, chopped
1 tbsp stuffing mix

Dry-fry the onion, leek, celery and mushrooms for 3–5 minutes until soft.

Place the potatoes in a large saucepan, cover with cold water and bring to the boil. Add the carrots and cook for 5 minutes. Add the cauliflower and gently boil until all the vegetables are just cooked. Drain, reserving the cooking liquid.

To make the white sauce, reserve 2 tablespoons of milk and heat the rest in a saucepan. Mix the reserved milk with the cornflour. Gradually whisk in the hot milk and 1/4 pint/5 fl oz (125 ml) of cooking liquid, stirring continuously. Return to the saucepan and cook until the sauce thickens. Add more cornflour if necessary. Season well.

Remove from the heat and stir in the parsley. Pour the sauce over the vegetables, mix and place in an ovenproof dish. Sprinkle over the stuffing mix and bake in a preheated oven at 180°C, 350°F, or Gas Mark 4 for 15 minutes.

Garnish with the parsley sprigs and tomato lily, and serve.

Vegetable Curry
(Serves 4)

3 oz (75 g) [dry weight] soya chunks or chopped tofu, or tinned vegetable protein
1 x 15 oz (375 g) can tomatoes
1 bay leaf
1 eating apple, cored and chopped
2 tsp oil-free sweet pickle
1 tsp tomato purée
1 medium onion, peeled and chopped
1 tbsp curry powder

Soak the soya chunks in 2 cups of boiling water for 10 minutes. Drain.

Place the soya chunks and all other ingredients in a saucepan and bring to the boil. Cover the saucepan and simmer for about 1 hour, stirring occasionally. If the mixture is too thin, remove the lid and cook on a slightly higher heat until the sauce reduces and thickens.

Serve on a bed of boiled brown rice (2 oz/50 g [dry weight] per person).

Vegetable and Herb Bake
(Serves 4)

$^1/_2$ pint/10 fl oz (250 ml) water
1 vegetable stock cube
1 x 8 oz (200 g) can chopped tomatoes
8 oz (200 g) carrots, trimmed, scraped and sliced
1 medium onion, peeled and chopped
1 large red pepper, deseeded and sliced
1 large courgette, sliced
4 sticks celery, chopped
4 oz (100 g) frozen peas
2 tsp dried basil
1 tsp tomato purée
salt and black pepper to taste
1 tbsp wholemeal flour
1 lb (400 g) potatoes, peeled and cooked
4 oz (100 g) Edam cheese, grated
2 tbsp semi-skimmed or skimmed milk
(in addition to allowance)
2 oz (50 g) wholemeal breadcrumbs
pinch paprika

Place the water, stock cube and tomatoes in a saucepan and bring to the boil. Add the carrots and simmer for 10 minutes. Add the onion, pepper, courgette, celery, peas, basil and tomato purée. Season well and simmer for a further 5–10 minutes.

Mix the flour with a little of the cooking liquid, and stir into the vegetable mixture to thicken.

Mash together the potatoes, cheese and milk. Spoon the vegetable mixture into a warm serving dish. Top with the potato mixture and sprinkle the breadcrumbs and a little paprika over. Grill until golden brown.

Serve with French bread (1 oz/25 g per person) and mixed salad.

Note: As this vegetarian dish is so low in fat, 1 oz (25 g) Edam cheese per person is permitted.

Vegetable Kebabs
(Serves 2)

1 green pepper, deseeded and chopped into $^3/_4$ inch
(2 cm) squares
1 red pepper, deseeded and chopped into $^3/_4$ inch
(2 cm) squares
1 large Spanish onion, peeled and cut into large
pieces *or* 6 oz (150 g) small button onions, peeled
8 oz (200 g) button mushrooms, washed
4 courgettes, coarsely sliced
1 lb (400 g) average-sized fresh tomatoes, sliced
across sideways
1 tsp thyme
cayenne pepper

Thread the vegetable pieces alternately on 4 skewers to make 4 kebabs.

Cover a baking sheet with aluminium foil and place the kebabs on the foil, sprinkling each kebab with thyme. Wrap the foil around the kebabs to make a parcel and cook in a preheated oven at 180°C, 350°F, or Gas Mark 4 for 35 minutes.

Remove from the oven. Unwrap and place kebabs on a bed of hot sweetcorn (4 oz/100 g) and boiled brown rice (2 oz/50 g [dry weight] per person), and sprinkle with cayenne pepper to taste. Replace in the oven for 1 minute.

Vegetable Risotto
(Serves 4)

6 oz (150 g) [dry weight] brown rice
1 large onion, peeled and chopped
1 green pepper, deseeded and finely chopped
1 red pepper, deseeded and finely chopped
1 tsp oregano
1 x 8 oz (200 g) can tomatoes
2 oz (50 g) mushrooms, sliced
1 wine glass white wine
2 oz (50 g) frozen peas
salt and black pepper to taste

Simmer the rice in salted water until it is half-cooked. Bring a fresh pint of water to the boil in another saucepan and add to the half-cooked rice.

Meanwhile, dry-fry the onion and peppers in a non-stick frying pan, together with the oregano. When the onion is soft and brown in colour, add the tomatoes, mushrooms, glass of wine and frozen peas and cook for a few more minutes. When the rice is almost cooked, drain it and stir it into the vegetable mixture. Add salt and pepper to taste.

Serve immediately.

Vegetarian Chilli con Carne
(Serves 4)

3 oz (75 g) [dry weight] soya savoury mince
1 x 15 oz (375 g) can tomatoes
2 bay leaves
1 large onion, peeled and chopped
1 tsp yeast extract
1 x 15 oz (375 g) can red kidney beans
1 tsp chilli powder (or to individual taste)
1 tsp garlic granules (optional)

Add 2 cups of boiling water to the soya mince and leave to soak for 10 minutes.

Place all ingredients in a saucepan, cover and leave to cook for 30 minutes. Remove the lid and continue cooking until the mixture reaches a fairly thick consistency.

Serve with boiled brown rice. Allow 2 oz/50 g (dry weight) per person.

Vegetarian Loaf
(Serves 4)

1 lb (400 g) medium tofu
8 fl oz (200 ml) bolognese sauce
(low-fat, vegetarian brand)
1 medium onion, peeled and finely chopped
1 green pepper, deseeded and chopped
1 clove garlic, peeled and crushed
1 tsp dried oregano
$^1/_2$ tsp dried basil
1 oz (25 g) oats
1 oz (25 g) wholemeal flour
salt and black pepper to taste

Very lightly oil or spray with a non-stick cooking spray a 4 x 8 inch (10 x 20 cm) tin.

Rinse and drain the tofu and place it in a large bowl with half the sauce. Add the chopped onion, pepper, garlic and herbs and mash well with a fork. Add the oats and wholewheat flour and mix well. Press the mixture into the prepared tin and press down firmly. Bake in the preheated oven at 180°C, 350°F, or Gas Mark 4 for 45 minutes.

Heat the remaining sauce ready to serve with the loaf. Allow the loaf to stand for 5 minutes before inverting on to a serving dish.

Serve with the hot sauce and unlimited vegetables.

VEGETABLE SIDE DISHES

Dry-roast Parsnips
(Serves 4)

4–6 medium-sized parsnips
salt

Peel and cut parsnips in half lengthways. Blanch in cold salted water and bring to the boil.

Drain thoroughly and sprinkle lightly with salt. Place on a non-stick baking tray, without fat, and bake in a preheated oven at 200°C, 400°F, or Gas Mark 6 for 30 minutes or until the parsnips are soft in the centre when pierced with a fork.

Dry-roast Potatoes

Choose medium potatoes of even size. Peel, then blanch them by putting into cold salted water and bringing to the boil.

Drain thoroughly. Lightly scratch the surface of each potato with a fork, and sprinkle lightly with salt.

Place on a non-stick baking tray, without fat, in a preheated oven at 200°C, 400°F, or Gas Mark 6 for about 1–1½ hours.

Potato and Parsley Bake
(Serves 4)

1¼ lb (500 g) potatoes, peeled and thickly sliced
8 oz (200 g) carrots, trimmed, scraped and cut into julienne strips
4 oz (100 g) parsley and thyme stuffing mix
grated zest and juice of 1 lemon
black pepper to taste
2 tsp sesame seeds
parsley sprigs to garnish

Place the potatoes in a saucepan with just enough cold water to cover. Bring slowly to the boil, add the carrots and cook gently for 5 minutes.

Make up the stuffing with boiling water to a moist consistency. Add the zest and 1 teaspoon of the lemon juice. Season with the black pepper.

Drain the vegetables reserving the cooking liquid. Layer half the potatoes into a lightly greased 7 inch (18 cm) ovenproof dish.

Spread half the stuffing over the potatoes and add the carrots.

Add the remaining stuffing and arrange the rest of the potato slices on top. Pour 3 fl oz (75 ml) of the cooking liquid over and sprinkle with sesame seeds.

Bake in a preheated oven at 180°C, 350°F, or Gas Mark 4 for 40–45 minutes until crisp and golden brown.

Garnish with parsley sprigs, and serve.

Ratatouille
(Serves 4)

1 small aubergine
1 tsp salt
1 large onion, peeled and thickly sliced
2 medium-sized courgettes (baby marrows), thickly sliced
1 small green pepper, deseeded and cut into strips
1 x 14 oz (350 g) can tomatoes
1 tbsp chopped fresh basil or 1 tsp dried basil
2 cloves garlic, peeled and crushed, or 1 tsp garlic paste
salt and black pepper to taste
a little extra chopped fresh basil to garnish

To make the ratatouille, cut the aubergine into 1 inch (2.5 cm) cubes, sprinkle 1 teaspoon salt over them and leave on a wire rack for 20–30 minutes. Then place in a colander and rinse well under cold running water.

Place all the vegetables, the tomatoes (including their juice), the fresh or dried basil and the garlic into a pan. Season to taste. Bring to the boil and simmer gently for 20–30 minutes, uncovered, until the vegetables are tender and most of the liquid has evaporated.

If chopped fresh basil is available, sprinkle a little over the top just before serving. Serve hot.

Savoury Carrots
(Serves 4)

1 lb (400 g) small carrots, trimmed and scraped
4 oz (100 g) onion, peeled and finely chopped
¼ pint/5 fl oz (12.5 ml) chicken stock
salt and black pepper to taste
chopped fresh parsley to garnish

Place all the ingredients except the parsley into a small saucepan. Bring to the boil and simmer until the stock has reduced and the vegetables are tender.

Drain, and sprinkle with chopped fresh parsley just before serving.

DESSERTS

Apple Meringue
(Serves 4)

2 Granny Smith cooking apples
6 oz (150 g) raspberries, fresh or frozen
5 egg whites
10 oz (250 g) caster sugar
8 oz (200 g) Wall's 'Too Good To Be True' ice cream (vanilla or strawberry)

Peel the apples and, using an apple corer, remove the core. Remove a thin slice from the base of each apple to make sure they will sit flat, then cut each apple in half across its centre so that the cavity can be filled.

Place on a microwave turntable and cook for 2 minutes on *full* power until slightly softened. Alternatively, cover with foil, place on a baking tray and cook in a moderate oven (180°C, 350°F, or Gas Mark 4) for 20 minutes.

Transfer the apples to a plate (ovenproof but not metal). Fill the cavity of each apple with raspberries. Leave to cool, and chill in the refrigerator for 30 minutes.

Whisk the egg whites until stiff peaks are formed, then continue whisking for a further minute while gradually adding the caster sugar.

Remove the apples from the refrigerator, place a scoop of ice cream on each and completely cover with the meringue mixture.

Bake in a preheated oven at 240°C, 475°F, or Gas Mark 9 for 4 minutes until the meringue is set and slightly browned. Serve immediately.

Note: Granny Smith apples make an ideal base in this recipe as they keep their crisp texture and really fresh flavour.

Apricot and Banana Fool

(Serves 4)

2 egg whites
10 drops liquid artificial sweetener
4 bananas
2 oz (50 g) dried apricots (the no-soak variety)
8 oz (200 g) low-fat Quark
mint leaves and slices of lemon or lime to garnish

Whisk the egg whites until they stand in peaks. Add the artificial sweetener.

Peel the bananas and mash them well in a bowl. Using a pair of scissors, snip the apricots into small pieces and add to the bananas. Mix with the Quark then gently fold into the beaten egg whites.

Divide into 4 individual dishes and chill until ready to serve. The fool is best served within 30 minutes.

Decorate each dish with a mint leaf or slice of lemon or lime.

Baked Banana

(Serves 1)

1 banana
pinch brown sugar
1 tbsp raisins
pinch cinnamon
4 tbsp water

Peel and slice the banana and place in a shallow dish. Sprinkle with the brown sugar, raisins and cinnamon. Pour the water over and bake at 180°C, 350°F, or Gas Mark 4 for 30 minutes.

For special occasions substitute rum for the water.

Baked Stuffed Apple

(Serves 1)

1 large cooking apple
1 oz (25 g) dried fruit
1 tsp honey
2 tbsp low-fat natural yogurt

Remove the core from the apple but leave the apple intact. Using a sharp knife, score around the 'waist' of the apple, cutting through only the skin.

Mix together the dried fruit and honey and pile into the cavity of the apple.

Place in an ovenproof dish and bake in a preheated oven at 200°C, 400°F, or Gas Mark 6 for about 30 minutes, or until cooked.

Serve with the yogurt spooned over the top.

Fresh Fruit Salad

(Serves 6–8)

zest and juice of 1 lemon and 2 oranges
$^1/_2$ pint/10 fl oz (250 ml) water
1 oz (25 g) sugar substitute (e.g. Canderel)
1 red apple, cored and thinly sliced
1 Granny Smith apple, cored and thinly sliced
1 large pear, chopped into $^1/_2$ inch (1 cm) pieces
2 oranges, peeled and segmented
black and green grapes, halved and deseeded
2 kiwi fruits, peeled and sliced
1 banana, peeled and sliced
8 oz (200 g) any seasonal soft fruit, e.g. strawberries, raspberries, cherries etc., but choose only one type

Place the zest of the lemon and oranges in a small pan with the water, bring to the boil, reduce the heat and simmer for 5 minutes. Remove from the heat and allow to cool.

Add the juice from the lemon and oranges to the pan, then add the sugar substitute. Stir well.

Place the fruit into a serving dish. Strain the syrup on to the fruit, mix well and stir to bring out the various flavours.

Note: The fruit salad will keep for 1–2 days in the refrigerator.

Fruit Brûlée

(Serves 4)

1 lb (400 g) prepared fruit (see below)
1–2 tbsp lemon juice
1 lb (400 g) low-fat fromage frais or yogurt
4–5 tbsp demerara or palm sugar

Any assortment of fruit can be used for this sweet. Oranges, grapes and apples form a good base; pears, plums, raspberries, strawberries and redcurrants all provide a contrast in flavour and texture. Even in winter a few frozen raspberries can be used, but frozen strawberries are not recommended as they are too moist.

Using a small serrated knife, peel the oranges and cut out the segments. Wash the grapes, cut them in half and remove the pips. Peel, core and dice the apples and pears and toss in the lemon juice. Remove the stones from the plums and cut into pieces. Wash the raspberries, strawberries and redcurrants. Drain all the fruit well so that it is quite dry. Place the fruit in a heatproof dish, and chill in the refrigerator.

Preheat the grill until it is very hot. Just before you place the dish under the grill, spread the fromage frais or yogurt over the fruit and sprinkle the sugar on top (it is important that this is done immediately before grilling, otherwise the sugar melts and does not caramelise). Place the dish as high under the grill as possible and watch it all the time to see that it caramelises evenly. Turn the dish, if necessary, and take care that the sugar does not burn.

Allow to cool, then chill before serving.

Fruit Sundae
(Serves 2)

8 oz (200 g) prepared fruit (blackberries, raspberries or strawberries, or a mixture)
6 drops liquid artificial sweetener
5 oz (125 g) low-fat natural yogurt
1 egg white
angelica and vermouth (optional)

Stir the fruit, sweetener and yogurt together thoroughly.

Whisk the egg white until stiff and fold into the fruit mixture.

Spoon into serving glasses. Top with angelica and vermouth if desired.

Hot Cherries
(Serves 2)

1 x 8 oz (200 g) can black cherries in syrup
2 fl oz (50 ml) cherry brandy (optional)
1 tsp arrowroot
4 oz (100 g) Wall's 'Too Good To Be True' ice cream

Strain the cherries, reserving the juice. Heat the juice in a pan. Add the cherry brandy (if used) and thicken with enough slaked arrowroot (approximately 1 tea-spoon mixed with water) to make a syrup. Pour over the ice cream.

Serve with the cherries immediately.

Kiwi Fruit Mousse
(Serves 2)

4 kiwi fruits
2 oz (50 g) low-fat soft cheese
1/2 level tsp paprika
black pepper to taste
1 tbsp lemon juice
1 tsp white wine vinegar
salt to taste

Remove both ends of each kiwi fruit with a sharp knife. Do not peel. Using an apple corer, carefully remove the centre of each fruit. Reserve. Mix together the cheese, paprika and black pepper. Fill the hollowed centres with the cheese mixture and place in a refrigerator to chill.

Chop the reserved fruit cores finely, and add the lemon juice and white wine vinegar. Mix the kiwi fruit dressing well with a fork, and season to taste.

Peel the filled kiwi fruits carefully. Cut each into 4 thick slices. Arrange on plates over the evenly distributed kiwi fruit dressing. Serve chilled.

Pears in Meringue
(Serves 6)

6 ripe dessert pears, peeled but left whole
1/2 pint/10 fl oz (250 ml) apple juice
3 egg whites
6 oz (150 g) caster sugar
4 tbsp low-fat fromage frais

Place the pears in a saucepan with the apple juice and cook until just tender. Cut a slice off the bottom of each pear to enable them to sit in a dish without falling over. Place them, well spaced out, in an ovenproof dish.

Whisk the egg whites in a large and completely grease-free bowl, preferably with a balloon whisk or rotary beater, as these make more volume than an electric whisk.

When the egg whites are firm and stand in peaks, whisk in 1 tablespoon of the caster sugar for 1 minute. Fold in the remainder of the sugar with a metal spoon, cutting the egg whites rather than mixing them.

Place the egg white and sugar mixture into a large piping bag with a metal nozzle (any pattern) and pipe a pyramid around each pear, starting from the base and working upwards. Place in a preheated oven and bake at 160°C, 325°F, or Gas Mark 3 until firm and golden.

Serve hot or cold with the fromage frais.

Kiwi Fruit Sorbet
(Serves 4)

5 kiwi fruits, peeled and thickly sliced
2 tbsp Cointreau
4 oz (100 g) caster sugar
1 egg white
fresh fruit to decorate

Place the kiwi fruits in a blender with the Cointreau and sugar, and purée. Pour the mixture into a bowl and freeze for about 2 hours.

Tip the mixture into a fresh bowl and whisk to break up the crystals. Beat the egg white until stiff and fold into the fruit purée. Place into a decorative bowl and freeze.

Remove from the freezer half an hour before serving. Decorate with fresh fruit of your choice.

Tropical Fruit Salad
(Serves 4)

1 mango
1 lb (400 g) water melon
3 passion fruits
3 bananas

Peel the mango and, using a teaspoon, scoop out any flesh left on the skin. Holding the mango over a bowl, cut into slices close to the stone. Cut the melon flesh into 1/2 inch (1 cm) cubes, discarding all the seeds. Halve the passion fruits and scoop out the flesh with a teaspoon.

Peel and slice the bananas. Mix all the fruit together in the bowl and chill lightly until ready to serve.

Serve within 30 minutes of preparing.

Low-fat Rice Pudding

(Serves 4)

$1^1/_2$ oz (37.5 g) short-grain rice
1 oz (25 g) sugar
1 pint/20 fl oz (500 ml) semi-skimmed and
skimmed milk (in addition to allowance)

Place all the ingredients into an ovenproof dish. Bake in a preheated oven at 150°C, 300°F, or Gas Mark 2 until the rice is soft.

Low-fat Trifle

(Serves 4)

1 packet sugar-free jelly
2 medium-sized bananas, peeled and sliced
1 x 17 oz (425 g) carton low-fat custard
2 x 5 oz (125 g) vanilla virtually fat-free yogurt

Make the jelly as instructed on the packet in a large dish. Add the bananas and leave to set.

When set, cover the jelly with the low-fat custard, then smooth the yogurt over the top.

Meringue Biscuits

(Makes approximately 30 biscuits)

4 egg whites
8 oz (200 g) caster sugar

Whisk the egg whites until they stand in stiff peaks. Add 1 oz (25 g) of the caster sugar and continue whisking for 1 minute. Fold in the remaining caster sugar.

Place the meringue mixture into a large piping bag with a large nozzle – any pattern nozzle will do. Gently pipe the egg whites into small pyramids on to a non-stick baking sheet. Place in a preheated oven and bake at 150°C, 300°F, or Gas Mark 2 for approximately 2 hours or until crisp and beige in colour. The meringues should easily come away from the baking sheet. If they don't, gently prise them off with a sharp, pliable knife.

Note: Meringues may be stored in an airtight container for up to 2 weeks.

Apple and Blackberry Cake

(Makes 10–12 slices)

1 cup All-Bran cereal
$^1/_2$ cup skimmed milk (in addition to allowance)
1 cup sugar
1 cup self-raising flour
1 cup grated Bramley apple
3 oz (75 g) blackberries

Soak the All-Bran in the milk for about 2 hours until soft.

Add the sugar, flour and grated apple, mixing well. Fold in the blackberries and pour into a lined 2 lb (800 g) loaf tin.

Bake in the centre of the oven for 2 hours at 150°C, 300°F, or Gas Mark 2.

Leave to cool. Slice when cold.

Banana and Sultana Cake

(1 serving = $^1/_2$ inch/1.25 cm slice)

1 lb 3 oz (475 g) ripe bananas (5 large), peeled
2 eggs, beaten
6 oz (150 g) brown sugar
4 oz (100 g) sultanas
8 oz (200 g) self-raising flour

Mash the bananas in a mixing bowl. Add the eggs, sugar and sultanas and mix the flour in. Place in a lined 2 lb (800 g) loaf tin or cake tin.

Bake for $1^1/_2$ hours in a preheated oven at 180°C, 350°F, or Gas Mark 4. Store in an airtight tin for 24 hours before serving. Suitable for freezing.

Note: This is an economical recipe as very ripe bananas can often be purchased cheaply.

Prune Cake

(Serves 8–10)

6 oz (150 g) self-raising flour
6 oz (150 g) caster sugar
3 eggs
1 heaped tsp mixed spice (cinnamon or ginger)
4 oz (100 g) stoned prunes,
soaked in tea overnight and drained
icing sugar (optional)

Place all the ingredients in a food processor, and mix well.

Pour the mixture into a lined and lightly greased rectanglular cake tin and bake in a preheated oven at 200°C, 400°F, or Gas Mark 6 for approximately 30–35 minutes. Remove from the oven and leave to cool in the tin.

While the cake is still warm pour a weak solution of icing sugar mixed with water over the top (if desired).

Note: You will find that this cake has a slight chewy texture to it.

Sultana Cake

(Serves 6)

$1^1/_2$ cups self-raising wholemeal flour
(fine stoneground)
$^3/_4$ cup Bran Flakes
$1^1/_2$ cups sultanas
$1^1/_2$ cups semi-skimmed or skimmed milk
(in addition to allowance)
apricot jam to spread

Mix the flour and Bran Flakes together in a bowl. Add the sultanas and mix well. Pour the milk into the mixture and stir well.

Bake in the oven in a non-stick muffin pan at 200°C, 400°F, or Gas Mark 6 for 5–8 minutes until cooked.

To serve, spread with a little apricot jam.

Swiss Roll Meringue

(Serves 6–8)

4 egg whites
6 oz (150 g) caster sugar
1 tsp vanilla essence
1 tbsp each icing sugar and caster sugar for sprinkling

Filling

12 oz (300 g) raspberries, puréed
1/2 pint/10 fl oz (250 ml) low-fat fromage frais
2 tsp gelatine dissolved in 2 tbsp hot water

Whisk the egg whites until stiff. Whisk in 3 oz (75 g) of the caster sugar, then fold in the remaining sugar and add the vanilla essence.

Line a large Swiss roll tin with baking parchment. Spread the meringue mixture evenly into the tin.

Bake in a preheated oven at 160°C, 325°F, or Gas Mark 3 for 12 minutes. Reduce the oven temperature to 150°C, 300°F, or Gas Mark 2 and bake for a further 15 minutes.

Tip the roulade carefully on to a separate sheet of baking parchment. Sprinkle liberally with the icing sugar and caster sugar. Leave to cool.

To make the filling, freeze two-thirds of the raspberry purée until forming crystals.

Beat the fromage frais and gelatine together. Leave to chill until the mixture starts to thicken and set.

Add the semi-frozen raspberry purée and then spread over the roulade. Roll up like a Swiss roll and freeze.

Serve with the remaining raspberry purée.

SAUCES AND DRESSINGS

Garlic and Yogurt Dressing

1 clove garlic, peeled and crushed
5 oz (125 g) low-fat natural yogurt
1 tbsp wine vinegar
1 tsp reduced-oil salad dressing
salt and black pepper to taste

Mix all the ingredients together. Store in a screw-top jar in the refrigerator and use within 2 days.

Oil-free Vinaigrette Dressing

3 tbsp white wine vinegar or cider vinegar
1 tbsp lemon juice
1/2 tsp black pepper
1/2 tsp salt
1 tsp sugar
1/2 tsp French mustard
chopped herbs (thyme, marjoram, basil or parsley)

Place all the ingredients in a container, seal, then shake well. Taste, and add more salt or sugar as desired.

Coleslaw

(Serves 4)

2 large carrots, trimmed and scraped
8 oz (200 g) white cabbage, trimmed
1 Spanish onion, peeled
4 oz (100 g) reduced-oil salad dressing

Wash the carrots and cabbage, then grate them and finely chop the onion. Mix together in a bowl with the reduced-oil dressing. Serve immediately or keep chilled and eat within 2 days.

Prawn Cocktail Sauce

(Serves 1)

1 tbsp tomato ketchup
1/2 tbsp reduced-oil salad dressing
1 tbsp low-fat natural yogurt
black pepper to taste
dash Tabasco sauce

Mix all the ingredients together and store in a screw-top jar in the refrigerator until required.

Maintaining your new figure

There are many benefits in following a low-fat diet. Not only do your taste buds change (many people find the taste of fatty food becomes repulsive and indigestible), but your general feeling of well-being and your energy levels are increased to such an extent that you often feel significantly younger than your years. Add to this the fact that you look so much better after losing the unwanted fat from the body – well, it's like being a brand new person – and you don't want to lose that sense of feeling on top of the world.

Having achieved your goal, it is obviously important to sustain it and, provided you don't slip back into your old, high-fat eating habits, this can be accomplished without too much difficulty. My simple golden rules for weight maintenance are as follows:

TEN TIPS FOR SUCCESSFUL WEIGHT MAINTENANCE

1   Always select low-fat alternatives and check the nutrition panel to ascertain the fat content of foods before you buy them.

2   Continue to eat a low-fat diet and never add fat while preparing or serving food. However, you may now add a few more dressings to salads and occasionally eat a little, low-fat hard cheese.

3   Eat as much as you like of low-fat foods at meal times. Continue to eat three meals a day, but avoid between-meal snacks. Nibbling between meals can seriously damage your waistline.

4   Continue to exercise regularly. This will not only keep your heart fitter, but it will also help keep your metabolic rate higher so that weight maintenance becomes easier.

5   Avoid temptation by not keeping biscuits and sweets (or, in fact, anything you think might tempt you in a weak moment) in the house. Instead, have plenty of fresh fruit available for you, your children and even the non-weight-conscious members of your family to consume. Also, fat-free cakes can soon become firm favourites with the family.

6   When dining out, enjoy yourself and by all means relax the rules a little, but try to be sensible when making your selection from the menu. It is easier to limit the damage than to cure the problem later.

7   Keep an eye on the scales and the tape measure. If you gain more than 2 lb (1 kg) in weight or more than 1 inch (2.5 cm) at any circumference, return to the diet for two days and your weight should return to normal. It is a great deal easier to lose one or two pounds than three or four!

8   Never skip a meal as this can lead to uncontrolled eating later. Also, please remember that it is important to eat breakfast every day as this helps to kick-start your metabolism.

9   The occasional dietary indiscretion is not the end of the world, but do remember that one lapse can lead to another. Before you know where you are, you may find yourself on a slippery slope and returning to your old eating habits – the ones that made you overweight in the first place – so indulge with caution!

10   Realise that weight maintenance is totally within your control. If you want to stay slim you can do so. Keep your 'before' photographs to hand, and each time you contemplate whether that cream cake really is worth it, look at those photographs.

Fat Content Chart

Grams per 25 g/1 oz (approx)

Food	Fat (g per 25 g/1 oz)
Alcohol	negligible
Beans	
Baked	negligible
Kidney	negligible
Biscuits	
Sweet	6
Savoury	5
Rye	1
Bread	1
Breakfast cereal	
Muesli type	3
Porridge (dry)	2
Flakes – corn or bran	1
Weetabix	1
Fats and oils	
Butter and margarine	20
Flora	20
Low fat spread	10
Gold Lowest	4
Oil – all types	25
Cakes	
Cakes – average	6
Pastry – average	9
Cheese	
Ordinary Cheddar	9
Low fat brands	5
Cream cheese	12
Low-fat soft cheese	2

● = negligible

Grams per 25 g/1 oz (approx)

	1	2	3	4	5	6	7	8	9	10	11	12	13	14	15	16	17	18	19	20	21	22	23	24	25
Fromage frais	██	██																							
Low-fat fromage frais	●																								
Cottage cheese	●																								
Quark – low fat	●																								

Confectionery

	1	2	3	4	5	6	7	8	9	10	11	12	13	14	15	16	17	18	19	20	21	22	23	24	25
Sweets – boiled/mint	●																								
Chocolate	██	██	██	██	██	██	██	██																	

Cream

	1	2	3	4	5	6	7	8	9	10	11	12	13	14	15	16	17	18	19	20	21	22	23	24	25
Single	██	██	██	██	██																				
Whipping	██	██	██	██	██	██	██	██	██	██															
Double	██	██	██	██	██	██	██	██	██	██	██	██													
Cornish clotted	██	██	██	██	██	██	██	██	██	██	██	██	██	██	██										

Eggs

	1	2	3	4	5	6	7	8	9	10	11	12	13	14	15	16	17	18	19	20	21	22	23	24	25
Whole	██	██	██																						
White only	●																								
Yolk only	██	██	██	██	██	██	██																		

Fish

	1	2	3	4	5	6	7	8	9	10	11	12	13	14	15	16	17	18	19	20	21	22	23	24	25
Fatty fish	██	██	██	██	██																				
White fish	██																								

Flour

	1	2	3	4	5	6	7	8	9	10	11	12	13	14	15	16	17	18	19	20	21	22	23	24	25
All types – average	██																								

Grains

	1	2	3	4	5	6	7	8	9	10	11	12	13	14	15	16	17	18	19	20	21	22	23	24	25
All types – average	██																								

Fruit

	1	2	3	4	5	6	7	8	9	10	11	12	13	14	15	16	17	18	19	20	21	22	23	24	25
Most types	●																								
Exceptions: Avocado	██	██	██	██	██	██																			

● = negligible

Grams per 25 g/1 oz (approx)

Food	1	2	3	4	5	6	7	8	9	10	11	12	13	14	15	16	17	18	19	20	21	22	23	24	25

Fruit continued

Food	Approx grams per 25 g/1 oz
Coconut flesh	~9.5
Olives	~3

Game

Food	Approx grams per 25 g/1 oz
Roast – without skin	~2

Ice cream

Food	Approx grams per 25 g/1 oz
Choc ice	~6.5
Plain	~3

Marzipan | ~6.5

Meat

Food	Approx grams per 25 g/1 oz
Bacon – lean only	~4.5
Bacon – lean & fat	~9
Beef – lean only	~2.5
Beef – lean & fat	~5
Lamb – lean only	~2.5
Lamb – lean & fat	~5.5
Pork – lean only	~2.5
Pork – lean & fat	~5.5
Sausages – average	~6.5
Salami	~10.5

Milk

Food	Approx grams per 25 g/1 oz
Fresh	~1.5
Skimmed	• (negligible)
Coffee whitener	~9

Nuts – average | ~15

Offal – average | ~2

● = negligible

Grams per 25 g/1 oz (approx)

	1	2	3	4	5	6	7	8	9	10	11	12	13	14	15	16	17	18	19	20	21	22	23	24	25

Pasta – average ● (negligible)

Pickles ● (negligible)

Poultry
Chicken – light meat – no skin — 1
Chicken – dark meat – no skin — 2
Duck – meat only – no skin — 3
Turkey – light meat ● (negligible)
Turkey – dark meat — 1

Puddings
Cheesecake — 9
Christmas pudding — 4
Fruit pie — 5
Jelly ● (negligible)
Meringues ● (negligible)
Pancakes — 5
Trifle — 2

Pulses & lentils ● (negligible)

Rice ● (negligible)

Sauces
Reduced-oil dressing — 4
Salad cream — 7
Mayonnaise — 16
French dressing — 19
Tomato ketchup ● (negligible)

Soups – average — 1

● = negligible

Grams per 25 g/1 oz (approx)

Food	Approx. fat (grams per 25 g/1 oz)
Soya	
Full fat	~7
Low fat	~2
Sugar	• (negligible)
Vegetables	
Most (including potatoes)	• (negligible)
Exceptions:	
Ackee	~5
Avocado	~7
Green mung beans	~2
Vegetables – cooked with fat	
Fried mushrooms	~6
Fried onions	~9
Potatoes – roast with fat	~2
Potatoes – chips (frozen & fried)	~5
Oven chips – frozen	~3
Crisps	~9
Yogurt	
Most low-fat brands	• (negligible)
French style set yogurt	• (negligible)
Yorkshire pudding	~3

• = negligible

WEIGHT AND INCH LOSS RECORD CHART

														Total loss
DATE:														
Weight														
Total weight lost to date														
Bust														
Waist														
Widest part														
Hips														
L. Thigh														
R. Thigh														
L. Knee														
R. Knee														
L. Arm														
R. Arm														
Total inches lost this week														
Total to date														

(To be completed 4 weeks after commencement of the plan)

1. *NAME:* MR/MRS/MISS/MS_____

Please print and underline surname

2. *ADDRESS:*_____

_____

_____

POSTCODE:_____

3. *AGE:* in which group do you belong: (Please tick)

1	☐ 15–24	5	☐ 55–64
2	☐ 25–34	6	☐ 65–74
3	☐ 35–44	7	☐ 75–84
4	☐ 45–54	8	☐ 85–94

4. *HEIGHT:* _____ ft _____ ins (m)

5. What did you weigh when you commenced the plan? _____ st _____ lb

6. What is your present weight? _____ st _____ lb

7. How would you have described yourself before you commenced this plan?

1	☐ very overweight	3	☐ slightly overweight
2	☐ quite overweight	4	☐ not overweight

8. For how many week have you followed the plan? _____ wks

9. How strictly did you follow this plan?

1 ☐ very strictly 2 ☐ moderately strictly 3 ☐ not very strictly

10. How much *weight* did you lose whilst on this plan? _____

11. How many inches did you lose from the following areas?

bust/chest	_____ inches	left thigh	_____ inches
waist	_____ inches	right thigh	_____ inches
abdomen	_____ inches	left knee	_____ inches
hips	_____ inches	right knee	_____ inches
widest part	_____ inches	left arm	_____ inches
		right arm	_____ inches

12. What are your present measurements in the following areas?

bust/chest	_____ inches	left thigh	_____ inches
waist	_____ inches	right thigh	_____ inches
abdomen	_____ inches	left knee	_____ inches
hips	_____ inches	right knee	_____ inches
widest part	_____ inches	left arm	_____ inches
		right arm	_____ inches

13. Which part of your body did you most want to reduce? (Tick more than one area if you wish)

1	☐ bust	5	☐ knees
2	☐ waist	6	☐ arms
3	☐ stomach	7	☐ other (please state): _____
4	☐ thighs		

14. On previous diet and/or exercise plans have you been able to reduce these areas?

1 ☐ No   2 ☐ Only a little

3 ☐ Yes. If I've lost weight I've lost it from these areas.

15. Are you surprised with your inch loss?

1 ☐ yes   2 ☐ not particularly   3 ☐ no

16. What is your reaction after following this plan?

1	☐ delighted with results	2	☐ pleasantly surprised
3	☐ satisfaction	4	☐ disappointment

17. What part of your body has reduced most significantly?

1	❑ bust	5	❑ thighs
2	❑ waist	6	❑ knees
3	❑ hips	7	❑ arms
4	❑ stomach	8	❑ other (please state):

_____

18. Do you think your cellulite (if you have any) has reduced?

1 ❑ yes   2 ❑ no   3 ❑ don't know

19. Do you feel healthier as a result of following the plan?

1 ❑ yes   2 ❑ no   3 ❑ no change

20. How did you find the plan affected your hair?

1 ❑ improved   2 ❑ deteriorated   3 ❑ same

21. How did you feel the plan affected your skin?

1 ❑ improved   2 ❑ deteriorated   3 ❑ same

22. How did you find the plan affected your nails?

1 ❑ improved   2 ❑ deteriorated   3 ❑ same

23. Did you experience any problems with constipation?

1 ❑ yes   2 ❑ no

24. Did you enjoy following the menus you selected?

1 ❑ yes   2 ❑ no

25. How often did you do the whole of the exercise plan?

1 ❑ every day   4 ❑ 1–2 times a week
2 ❑ almost every day   5 ❑ I didn't
3 ❑ 3–4 times a week

26. How often did you do the toning exercises?

1 ❑ every day   4 ❑ 1–2 times a week
2 ❑ almost every day   5 ❑ I didn't
3 ❑ 3–4 times a week

27. Have the exercises made a difference to:

your fitness 1 ❑ yes   2 ❑ no   3 ❑ don't
level   know
your shape 4 ❑ yes   5 ❑ no   6 ❑ don't
                                      know

28. Did you feel hungry?

1 ❑ often   3 ❑ hardly ever
2 ❑ occasionally   4 ❑ never

29. Before embarking on the diet plan did you ever have an eating binge?

1 ❑ often   2 ❑ occasionally   3 ❑ never

30. Did you binge at all on this diet plan?

1 ❑ often   2 ❑ occasionally   3 ❑ never

31. Did you binge less on this diet plan than with previous diets?

1 ❑ yes   2 ❑ about the same   3 ❑ no

32. Did you consume your alcohol allowance as specified within the diet plan?

1 ❑ yes   2 ❑ occasionally   3 ❑ no

33. Had you been on a diet just prior to following this diet?

1 ❑ yes   2 ❑ no

34. How would you describe your dieting history?

1 ❑ This was the first diet
2 ❑ I have only dieted very occasionally
3 ❑ I have tried more diets than I care to remember

35. Were you more successful following this diet than with previous diets?

1 ❑ yes   2 ❑ no

36. If `yes' was this because: (tick more than one if you wish)

1 ❑ it was easier to follow
2 ❑ it involved no calorie counting
3 ❑ it offered more freedom of choice
4 ❑ it was different from any diet I had tried before
5 ❑ I could have a drink and not feel guilty
6 ❑ I could eat so much more than on most diets

37. Have you enjoyed any health benefits as a result of following this plan?

1 ❑ yes   2 ❑ no

If the answer is yes, please give details below

_____

_____

Thank you for completing this questionnaire. I would be most grateful if you would make any further comments regarding the plan and how it may have affected you, particularly with regard to your health. Please write your comments on a separate piece of paper:

'I give Rosemary Conley permission to use the information given within this questionnaire in any subsequent book, publication or television series.'

Signed _____ Date _____

1 Please do not quote my name
2 Please use my initials only
3 You may use my name _(Please delete as appropriate)_
(N.B. Addresses will not be quoted but your town or country may be.)

Please return this form to Rosemary Conley, Rosemary Conley Diet & Fitness Clubs, Quorn House, Meeting Street, Quorn, Loughborough, Leicestershire LE12 8EX.
If you require a reply, please enclose sae.

Index of Recipes

American Turkey Burgers 160
Apple and Blackberry Cake 178
Apple Meringue 175–6
Apricot and Banana Fool 176
Apricot-glazed Chicken 162

Baked Banana 176
Baked Haddock 167
Baked Stuffed Apple 176
Banana and Sultana Cake 178
Basil, Chilli and Chicken Stir-fry 163
beef
    Beef Bourguignon 161
    Beef Casserole 161
    Beefburger in Bun 160
    Spaghetti Bolognese 161
Blackeye Bean Casserole 169–70
Broccoli Delight 170

Cabbage and Leek Bake 170
Campfire Kidneys 161
Carrot and Tarragon Soup 157–8
Cheesy Pears 156
chicken
    Apricot-glazed Chicken 162
    Basil, Chilli and Chicken Stir-fry 163
    Chicken Chasseur 163
    Chicken Chop Suey 163
    Chicken Dhansak 163
    Chicken with Herby Lemon Sauce 163
    Chicken Korma 163–4
    Chicken Liver Pâté with Brandy 156

Chicken Madras 164
Chicken and Mushroom Bake 164
Chicken Paprika 164
Chicken Provencale with Peppers and Onions 164
Chicken Risotto 165
Chicken and Sweetcorn Soup 158
Chilli Chicken 165
Chinese Chicken with Pineapple 165
Coq au Vin 165
Fruit and Chicken Salad 160
Jacket Potato with Curried Chicken and Yogurt Topping 160
Stir-fry Chicken in Black Bean Sauce 165
Tandoori Chicken Thatch 165–6
Tarragon Chicken 166
Tarragon Chicken Salad 166
Spicy Sweet and Sour Chicken or Pork with Crispy Vegetables 166
Sweet and Sour Chicken or Prawns with Crispy Vegetables 166
Chickpea and Fennel Casserole 170
Chilli Chicken 165
Chinese Apple Salad 160
Chinese Chicken with Pineapple 165
Chinese Menu 1 162
Chinese Menu 2 162

Chunky Vegetable Soup 158
Cod, Bacon, Cheese and Onion Bake 167
Cod in Parsley Sauce 168
Coleslaw 179
Coq au Vin 165
Cream of Leek and Potato Soup 158
Creamy Vegetable Soup 158–9
Crispy Garlic Mushrooms 156
Cullercoats Pie 168
Curried Chickpeas 170–1

desserts
    Apple and Blackberry Cake 178
    Apple Meringue 175–6
    Apricot and Banana Fool 176
    Baked Banana 176
    Baked Stuffed Apple 176
    Banana and Sultana Cake 178
    Fresh Fruit Salad 176
    Fruit Brûlée 176–7
    Fruit Sundae 177
    Hot Cherries 177
    Kiwi Fruit Mousse 177
    Kiwi Fruit Sorbet 177
    Low–fat Rice Pudding 178
    Low–fat Trifle 178
    Meringue Biscuits 178
    Pears in Meringue 177
    Prune Cake 178
    Sultana Cake 178
    Swiss Roll Meringue 179
    Tropical Fruit Salad 177

dressings
    Oil-free Vinaigrette Dressing 179
    Coleslaw 179
    Garlic and Yogurt Dressing 179
    Prawn Cocktail Sauce 179
Dry-roast Parsnips 175
Dry-roast Potatoes 175

fish
    Baked Haddock 167
    Cod, Bacon, Cheese and Onion Bake 167
    Cod in Parsley Sauce 168
    Cullercoats Pie 168
    Marinated Haddock 157
    Mediterranean Tuna Lasagne 168
    Melon and Prawn Salad 157
    Mussels in White Wine 157
    Trout Parcels with Dill Sauce 168
    Trout and Spinach Salad 169
    Tuna, Mushroom and Pasta Serenade 169
    Tuna and Sweetcorn Cakes 169
    Tuna Pasta with Tomatoes 169
French Tomatoes 156
Fresh Fruit Salad 176
Fruit and Chicken Salad 160
Fruit Brûlée 176–7
Fruit Sundae 177

Garlic and Mint Yogurt Dip with Crudités 157

Garlic and Yogurt Dressing 179
Grilled Grapefruit 157

Haricot Bean and Vegetable Soup 159
Hot Cherries 177

Jacket Potato with Curried Chicken and Yogurt Topping 160
Jacket Potato with Onion Mushrooms 160

Kiwi Fruit Mousse 177
Kiwi Fruit Sorbet 177

Lamb Kebabs with Onion Sauce 161
Low–fat Rice Pudding 178
Low–fat Trifle 178

Marinated Haddock 157
Mediterranean Tuna Lasagne 168
Melon and Prawn Salad 157
Meringue Biscuits 178
Mixed Bean Hotpot 171
Mussels in White Wine 157

Oil-free Vinaigrette Dressing 179
Orange and Grapefruit Cocktail 157
Oriental Vegetable Soup 159

Pears in Meringue 177
pork
    Pork Casserole 167

Spicy Sweet and Sour Chicken or Pork with Crispy Vegetables 166
Sweet and Sour Pork 166
Tasty Pork with Pasta 167
Potato and Parsley Bake 175
Potato and Watercress Soup 159
Prawn Cocktail Sauce 179
Prune Cake 178

Quorn Bolognese 171

Ratatouille 175

salads
    Chinese Apple Salad 160
    Fruit and Chicken Salad 160
    Melon and Prawn Salad 157
    Tarragon Chicken Salad 166
    Trout and Spinach Salad 169
    Yogurt Salad 172
Savoury Carrots 175
Souffle Potato and Ham Bake 167
soups
    Carrot and Tarragon Soup 157–8

Chicken and Sweetcorn Soup 158
Chunky Vegetable Soup 158–9
Cream of Leek and Potato Soup 158
Creamy Vegetable Soup 158
Haricot Bean and Vegetable Soup 159
Oriental Vegetable Soup 159
Potato and Watercress Soup 159
Tomato and Orange Soup 159
Watercress Soup 159
Spaghetti Bolognese 161
Spiced Bean Casserole 171
Spiced Turkey 165
Spicy Sweet and Sour Chicken or Pork with Crispy Vegetables 166
starters
    Cheesy Pears 156
    Chicken Liver Pâté with Brandy 156
    Crispy Garlic Mushrooms 156
    French Tomatoes 156
    Garlic and Mint Yogurt Dip with Crudites 157

Grilled Grapefruit 157
Orange and Grapefruit Cocktail 157
Marinated Haddock 157
Melon and Prawn Salad 157
Mussels in White Wine 157
Stir-fry Chicken in Black Bean Sauce 165
Stuffed Marrow 171–2
Stuffed Pitta Bread with Yogurt 172
Sultana Cake 178
Sweet and Sour Chicken or Prawns with Crispy Vegetables 166
Sweet and Sour Pork 166
Swiss Roll Meringue 179

Tandoori Chicken Thatch 165–6
Tarragon Chicken 166
Tarragon Chicken Salad 166
Tasty Pork with Pasta 167
Tofu Burgers 172
Tomato and Orange Soup 159
Tropical Fruit Salad 177
Trout Parcels with Dill Sauce 168
Trout and Spinach Salad 169
Tuna, Mushroom and Pasta Serenade 169

Tuna Pasta with Tomatoes 169
Tuna and Sweetcorn Cakes 169
turkey
    American Turkey Burgers 160
    Spiced Turkey 165

vegetables and vegetarian
    Blackeye Bean Casserole 169–70
    Broccoli Delight 170
    Cabbage and Leek Bake 170
    Chickpea and Fennel Casserole 170
    Curried Chickpeas 170–1
    Chunky Vegetable Soup 158
    Cream of Leek and Potato Soup 158
    Creamy Vegetable Soup 158–9
    Dry-roast Parsnips 175
    Dry-roast Potatoes 175
    Haricot Bean and Vegetable Soup 159
    Jacket Potato with Onion Mushrooms 160
    Mixed Bean Hotpot 171
    Oriental Vegetable Soup 159

Potato and Parsley Bake 175
Quorn Bolognese 171
Ratatouille 175
Savoury Carrots 175
Spiced Bean Casserole 171
Stuffed Marrow 171–2
Tofu Burgers 172
Vegetable Casserole 173
Vegetable Chilli 173
Vegetable Chop Suey 173
Vegetable Crunch 173
Vegetable Curry 173
Vegetable and Fruit Curry 172
Vegetable and Herb Bake 174
Vegetable Kebabs 174
Vegetable Risotto 174
Vegetarian Chilli con Carne 174
Vegetarian Loaf 174–5

Watercress Soup 159

Yogurt Salad 172